Jane Jackson, M.D.

CURRENT CLINICAL STRATEGIES

PSYCHIATRY

Lisa Burwell Sipes

Paul D. Chan

Preface

Current Clinical Strategies Guide to Psychiatric Diagnosis covers topics in psychiatry useful to medical students, residents and other health professionals. This manual provides a quick and convenient guide to the diagnosis and management of psychiatric disorders. All practitioners will find this book to be a vital asset, as psychiatric patients are encountered in all settings and in all specialties of medical practice.

This manual is structured to allow the clinician to individualize patient care by selecting a diagnosis based upon clinical indications, and then to choose the clinically indicated treatment plan from the alternatives provided.

Publishing information for authors may be obtained by writing to:

Current Clinical Strategies Publishing International
4200 Park Newport Ave., Suite 214
Newport Beach, California, USA 92660-6025
Phone or FAX: 714-721-0710

Printed in USA

ISBN 0-9626030-7-4

CONTENTS

ASSESSMENT AND EVALUATION

HISTORY:

Developmental history: Age of walking, talking, any delays.

Adolescent history: Extent of interpersonal relationships; substance abuse; school performance; parental problems; delinquency.

Adult History: Education, occupational and marital history; number of children, substance abuse.

Family History: History of psychiatric illness, suicide, alcohol or substance abuse.

Psychiatric and Medical History: Major physical illnesses, medication use (including over the counter medications). Psychiatric disorders, hospitalizations.

Current Problem and Stressors: Reason for consultation. Time of onset of problem; previous psychiatric treatment. Major stressors, (loss of employment, death of loved one, divorce, illness).

MENTAL STATUS EXAMINATION:

GENERAL APPEARANCE: Grooming, hygiene, clothing, posture, unusual physical characteristics.

ATTITUDE: Ability to interact well with interviewer; ability to establish eye contact; is the patient apathetic, cooperative, negative, positive, hostile, seductive.

SPEECH: Rate, tone, fluency, vocabulary. **Rapid pressured speech**: Speech that is rapid and difficult to interrupt. **Aphasia**: Inability to speak or comprehend language. **Dysarthria**: Poor articulation. **Poverty of Content**: Speech conveying little information. **Clanging**: Illogical speech based on sound rather than logical connections (rhyming, punning). **Derailment**: Speech that stops and resumes on a different topic. **Neologism**: Words invented by the patient.

THOUGHT PROCESS: **Blocking:** Sudden interruption of train of thought. **Flight of ideas**: Accelerated thought that jumps between ideas. **Loosening of Associations:** Illogical shifting between topics. **Tangentiality**: Thought which wanders from the original point. **Circumstantiality**: Unnecessary digression which eventually reaches the point. **Echolalia**: Echoing of words and phrases. **Perseveration**: Repetition of phrases or words in the flow of speech.

BEHAVIOR AND PSYCHOMOTOR ACTIVITY: Psychomotor agitation (restlessness, hyperactivity, hand wringing, pacing), psychomotor retardation (lack of facial expression less face, slowed speech, movement and thought); outbursts of anger, impulsiveness; sleep disturbances.

AFFECT: External range of expression observed by interviewer; blunted (extreme reduction in affect), restricted (mild reduction in affect), flat (absence of all or most affect), labile (sudden, multiple changes in affect), broad (wide range of affect), appropriate or inappropriate.

MOOD: Subjective, internal emotional tone of patient; depressed, elevated, expansive, anxious, irritable, angry, hopeless, euphoric.

THOUGHT CONTENT: **Obsessions:** Intrusive undesired ideas, images or impulses. **Paranoia:** False belief that others are trying to cause harm. **Delusion:** False, firmly held unshakable ideas. **Grandiosity:** Inflated sense of self worth. **Ideas of Reference:** Belief that people or events have specific, usually derogatory meaning for the patient. **Mood Congruent Concerns:** Concerns consistent with mood i.e., manic (grandiosity), depressed (guilt, worthlessness, inadequacy); phobias, suicidal or homicidal thoughts.

PERCEPTION:

Hallucinations: False sensory perceptions (auditory, gustatory, somatic, tactile, visual).

Illusions: Misinterpretations of reality (Mistaking shadows for monsters, hot air balloons for UFO's ext.)

Depersonalization: Feelings of unrealness as if one is outside ones body and observing.

Derealization: Feelings of unrealness involving the outer environment.

JUDGMENT/INSIGHT: Ability to make sound decisions regarding everyday activities. Insight into problems and understanding consequences of actions.

ATTENTION/CONCENTRATION:

Digit Span: Repeat five digits forward and backwards.

Spelling Forward/Backwards: Spell a five letter word forward then backwards.

Serial Sevens: Consecutively subtract sevens from 100.

ORIENTATION: Age, name, birth date, address, time, date, day, season, month, year, place, hospital, reason for being there.

Memory: Ability to memorize three objects for five minutes. Past five presidents.

General Knowledge: Ability to name the president, five large cities. current news events.

PSYCHOLOGICAL TESTING

Rorschach Test: The patient describes inkblots; this test assesses thinking patterns, personality functioning, ego-boundaries.

Minnesota Multiphasic Personality Inventory (MMPI): Battery of questions assessing personality characteristics. Results are given in ten scales: hypochondriasis, psychopathy, hysteria, social introversion, hypomania, paranoia, depression, schizophrenia, masculinity-femininity, psychasthenia anxiety/guilt/worry/phobias).

Thematic Apperception Test: A test consisting of ten cards with human figure drawings; patients are asked to make up a story for each card. This test provides information about intellect, fears, motivation, fantasies and interpersonal life.

Draw a Person Test: Patients draw a picture of a person, and then a picture of another person of the opposite sex of the first picture. The patient is asked about characteristics of each figure.

Sentence Completion Test: Patients are asked to complete sentences; provides insight into fears and preoccupations of the patient.

Wechsler Adult Intelligence Scale (WAIS): Measures performance, verbal and combined intelligence.

Laboratory Studies To Rule Out Physical Conditions: CBC, thyroid function tests, vitamin B-12 and folate levels, blood chemistry, blood alcohol level, urinalysis and drug screen, EEG, MRI.

SIGNS OF NEUROLOGICAL DISEASE

Agnosia: Loss of ability to recognize sensory stimuli.
Agraphia: Loss of ability to express thoughts in writing.
Alexia: Loss of ability to understand written language.
Aphasia: Disturbance in the ability to speak or comprehend language.
Apraxia: Loss of ability to carry out movements.
Dysarthria: Poor articulation of speech

MULTI-AXIAL SYSTEM OF CLASSIFICATION

Axis I: Current clinical diagnosis
Axis II: Developmental disorders or personality disorders
Axis III: Medical conditions
Axis IV: Severity of psychosocial stressors

Axis V: Global assessment of functioning

SELF TEST #1

1. **Blocking** is characteristic of a disturbance in:
   A) Thought content
   B) Perception
   • C) Speech or thought process
   D) Judgment
2. **Neologism** is a term used to describe:
   A) Speech that is based on association of sounds.
   B) Illogical shifting of topics which have no relation to one another.
   C) Difficulty in articulating words.
   • D) Use of words which are invented by the patient.
3. **Tangentiality** is a term used to describe:
   • A) Speech that wanders from its original point.
   B) Interruption of speech or train of thought.
   C) Lack of speech.
   D) Phrases or words which are repeated.
4. **Labile affect** is characterized by
   A) Normal range of affective expression.
   • B) Sudden, multiple changes in affective expression.
   C) Inappropriate affective expression.
   D) Absence of all or most affective expression.
5. **Delusions** are characteristic of a disturbance in:
   A) Mood
   • B) Thought content
   C) Affect
   D) Thought process
6. **Mood** is best defined as:
   A) Behavior and psychomotor activity
   • B) Internal feelings
   C) External expression of feelings.
   D) Ability to think clearly and make rational decisions.

ANSWERS TO SELF TEST #1

1. The answer is D. **Blocking** is a disturbance in thought process evident in speech.
2. The answer is D. **Neologism** is a the use of words that are invented by the patient.
3. The answer is A. **Tangentiality** is a term used to describe speech that wanders from its original point.
4. The answer is B. **Labile affect** is characterized by sudden, multiple changes in affective expression.
5. The answer is B. **Delusions** are a characteristic of a disturbance in thought content.
7. The answer is B. **Mood** is best defined as the patients internal feelings.

AFFECTIVE DISORDERS

MAJOR DEPRESSION

Definition: An affective disorder characterized by profound sadness and at least five of the following are required for diagnosis: depressed mood or anhedonia, sleep disturbances, fatigue, weight change, psychomotor retardation or agitation, suicidal ideation, thoughts of dying, difficulty concentrating, guilt or feelings of worthlessness.

Appearance: Sadness; blank; expressionless face; stooped posture, poor grooming.

Behavior and psychomotor activity: Anhedonia (loss of interest in usual activities), suicide attempts, social withdrawal, psychomotor agitation or retardation, lack of energy, change in appetite, weight loss or gain, hypersomnia, insomnia, impaired concentration and memory; somatic complaints, decreased libido, anxiety, irritability.

Speech: Soft or slowed speech, poverty of speech.

Mood: Depression, dysphoria (hopelessness, sadness).

Affect: Restricted affect (reduced range of emotions).

Perception: Psychotic features may be present, either mood congruent (depressive themes) or mood incongruent (delusions of reference, thought insertion).

Thought process: Slowed thought processes, delayed response to questions.

Thought Content: Suicidal ideation, thoughts of death, feelings of hopelessness, worthlessness, guilt, self reproach; possible delusions (poverty, persecutory), obsessive rumination.

Judgment: May be impaired due to feelings of hopelessness or delusional material.

Cognition: Distractibility, poor concentration.

Types of Depression:

Bipolar: One or more depressive episodes along with one or more manic episodes.

Unipolar: Depression alone.

Secondary: Depression secondary to other illness.

Endogenous/Primary: Depression without an identifiable cause.

Exogenous/Reactive: Depression with an identifiable cause.

Etiology/Predisposing Factors: Psychological, genetic, biological factors; depletion of serotonin or norepinephrine, endocrine factors.

Differential Diagnosis: Bereavement, adjustment disorder, dementia, reaction to physical illness, anxiety, schizophrenia, bipolar disorder, drug side effect, Addison's disease, anemia, Cushing's syndrome, hypothyroidism, hyperthyroidism, mononucleosis, nutritional deficiencies, electrolyte imbalances, Parkinson's disease, stroke, tumors.

Treatment: Rule out medical causes; psychotherapy, antidepressants, electroconvulsive therapy, antipsychotics for depressive psychosis.

DYSTHYMIA

Definition: Two year period of chronic depression not severe enough to meet the diagnostic criteria for major depression.

Behavior and psychomotor activity: Feelings of hopelessness, low self-esteem, anhedonia (inability to experience pleasure), difficulty concentrating, self destructive behavior, drug use, suicide attempts, sleep or appetite disturbances, fatigue, decreased libido.

Speech: Soft or slowed speech; poverty of speech.

Mood: Depressed.

Affect: Restricted affect (limited expression of emotion).

Thought Process: Slightly slowed thought process.

Thought Content: Feelings of hopelessness or worthlessness.

Etiology/Predisposing Factors: Psychological, genetic, biological factors; imbalances in serotonin or norepinephrine.

Treatment: Psychotherapy, behavior modification, antidepressants.

CYCLOTHYMIA

Definition: At least two years with periods of depression and elation not severe enough to meet the criteria for bipolar disorder.

Signs/Symptoms: Recurrent depressive and hypomanic episodes.

Etiology/Predisposing Factors: Genetic, biologic or psychological factors.

Differential Diagnosis: Bipolar disorder, borderline personality disorder, conduct disorder, attention deficit hyperactive disorder.

Treatment: Lithium, carbamazepine, antidepressants.

BIPOLAR DISORDER

Definition: At least one manic episode and one or more depressive episodes. he main feature of a manic episode is an irritable or elevated mood causing impairment in functioning, also known as Manic depression.

Appearance: Unusual, disheveled; flamboyant dress, excessive jewelry.

Behavior and psychomotor activity: Desire to socialize, increased goal directed activity, psychomotor agitation, low frustration tolerance; excessive involvement in multiple activities, hyperactivity, restlessness, social intrusiveness, irritability; inflated sense of self esteem; insomnia , distractibility, inability to concentrate, impulsiveness, increased or decreased appetite, engagement in reckless activities i.e., reckless driving, unwise spending, promiscuous sexual activity (increased libido), dramatic expression.

Speech: Talkative, rapid pressured speech (loud, quick and excessive), joking, clanging (speech dominated by sound).

Mood: Elevated, expansive, euphoric, irritable.

Affect: Labile affect (abrupt fluctuations of emotion).

Perception: Possible psychotic features, mood congruent (grandiose) or mood incongruent (reference, thought insertion).

Thought process: Flight of ideas (ideas on many different subjects in rapid succession), confusion.

Thought Content: Possible delusions of grandeur, excessive optimism.

Judgment: Impaired judgment.

Etiology/Predisposing Factors: Genetic and biologic factors.

Differential Diagnosis: Cyclothymia; cocaine or amphetamine intoxication, attention deficit disorder, schizophrenia, organic mood syndrome, dementia, multiple sclerosis.

Treatment: Psychotherapy, lithium, carbamazepine, valproic acid, antipsychotics, electroconvulsive therapy.

SELF TEST #5

1. All of the following are common symptoms of major depression except:
   A) Anhedonia
   B) Lack of energy.
   C) Flight of ideas.
   D) Slowed thought process.
2. All to the following symptoms are commonly seen in Dysthymia except:
   A) Self destructive behavior.
   B) Restricted affect.
   C) Rapid pressured speech.
   D) Feelings of hopelessness.
3. Your patient presents with grandiosity, hyperactivity, rapid pressured speech, clanging, flight of ideas and impaired judgement, the most likely diagnosis is;
   A) Brief reactive psychosis
   B) Manic episode
   C) Depressive episode
   D) Panic attack
4. The following symptoms are common during a manic episode except:
   A) Flat affect
   B) Delusions of Grandeur
   C) Hypersomnia
   D) Increase in goal directed activity

ANSWERS TO SELF TEST #5

1. The answer is C. **Flight of ideas** is not commonly seen in major depression.
2. The answer is C. **Rapid pressured speech** is not commonly seen in dysthymia.
3. The answer is B. Grandiosity, rapid pressured speech, clanging, flight of ideas, and impaired judgement are all common in **manic episodes.**
4. The answer is A. **Flat** affect is not commonly seen in manic episodes.

PSYCHOTIC DISORDERS

SCHIZOPHRENIA

Definition: A psychotic disorder characterized by disorganized thought process and deterioration in functioning and consisting of an Active (psychotic) phase and a residual phase (functioning below normal level), six months duration of illness.

Appearance: Unkept clothing, poor grooming, bizarre dress.

Behavior and psychomotor activity: Bizarre or inappropriate behavior, agitation, social isolation, deterioration in functioning, lack of initiative and motivation, identity disturbances, sensitivity, stereotyped behavior (repetition of a certain behavior), negativism (lack of cooperation); impulsive, unpredictable behavior, anhedonia (inability to experience pleasure), somatic complaints.

Speech: Word salads (stringing together of words that have no logical association), poverty of content (speech that conveys little information), echolalia (repeating of words or phrases), perseveration (words are repeatedly present in the flow of speech), mutism, neologisms (new words invented by the patient), excessive use of symbolism which may require interpretation.

Mood: Anxiety, anger, fearfulness, dysphoric mood and depression are all common. Patient may experience uncommon emotions i.e.; omnipotence, exaltation.

Affect: Emotional blunting, flat, inappropriate affect i.e., laughing and smiling during a sad experience.

Perception: Auditory or command hallucinations, visual, tactile, gustatory, olfactory, and somatic hallucinations. Depersonalization (feeling as if one is outside of oneself); derealization (feelings of unrealness involving external environment).

Thought process: Disorganized, illogical thinking; blocking (interruptions in train of thought), loosening of associations (ideas shift illogically from one topic to another), circumstantiality (thought containing digression before reaching a point), tangentiality (thought which wanders from the original point), flight of ideas (accelerated thought that jumps from idea to idea), verbigeration (illogical repetition).

Thought Content: Delusions of being controlled by an outside force, thought insertion (belief that thoughts are being inserted into one's mind), withdrawal (belief that thoughts are being removed from one's mind) or thought broadcasting (belief that others can read one's mind or hear one's thoughts), delusions of grandeur and persecution; religious, nihilistic and somatic delusions; ideas of reference (people or objects take on a significant, usually derogatory meaning to the patient), excessive fantasizing, distorted body image, fear, hypochondriacal concerns; use of defense mechanisms such as projection and denial.

Judgment: Impaired, may act on delusions or obey command hallucinations.

Cognition: Impaired.

Etiology/Predisposing Factors: Genetic predisposition; excess dopamine activity. Persons with withdrawn, eccentric, passive, impulsive schizotypal and schizoid personalities are more prone to develop schizophrenia.

CLASSIFICATION OF SCHIZOPHRENIA:

Paranoid Schizophrenia: Delusions of persecution or grandeur, hallucinations related to a single paranoid theme, aggressiveness, hostility.

Disorganized Schizophrenia: Loosening of associations, grimacing, delusions; flat, blunted or inappropriate affect; disorganized behavior, incoherence.

Excited Catatonic Schizophrenia: Psychomotor agitation, outbursts of anger.

Withdrawn Catatonic Schizophrenia: Catatonic posturing (bizarre or unusual postures), rigidity, stupor, mutism and negativism (resistance to all instructions or attempts to be moved). The patient is unresponsive to the environment or stimuli, but is aware of surroundings.

Undifferentiated Schizophrenia: Meets none of the above criteria for disorganized, catatonic or paranoid schizophrenia. Signs of psychosis may be present (delusions, hallucinations, incoherence).

Differential Diagnosis of Schizophrenia:

Brain injury or disease: Brain trauma, embolism, encephalitis, epilepsy (especially temporal lobe epilepsy), ischemia, tumor, pituitary adenoma.

Systemic Disease: AIDS dementia complex, Huntington's disease, hepatic encephalopathy, hyperthyroidism, hypoglycemia, lead poisoning, lupus, multiple sclerosis, syphilis, uremia, vasculitis, Wilson's disease.

Vitamin Deficiency: Vitamin B-12, B-6, folate, pyridoxine, thiamine, nicotinic acid deficiencies.

Psychiatric Disorders: Delirium, dementia, delusional disorder, bipolar disorder with psychotic features, mood disorder with psychotic features, schizoaffective or schizophreniform disorder.

Drugs Associated With A Schizophrenia Like Psychoses: Alcohol withdrawal, amphetamines, atropine, carbon monoxide, clonidine, cocaine, diazepam, disulfiram, ephedrine, hallucinogens, isoniazid, levodopa, lidocaine, lysergic acid (LSD), methamphetamine, phencyclidine (PCP), propoxyphene (Darvon), anticholinergic, sympathomimetics, sedatives.

Treatment: Antipsychotics, benzodiazepines for associated anxiety, psychotherapy.

SCHIZOPHRENIFORM DISORDER: Same as schizophrenia except duration of less than six months.

SCHIZOAFFECTIVE DISORDER: Symptoms of schizophrenia along with mood symptoms.

BRIEF REACTIVE PSYCHOSIS

Definition: Psychotic episode with abrupt onset after major stressor, duration of less than six months.

Appearance: Eccentric appearance; unusual, unkept clothing.

Behavior and Psychomotor Activity: Unusual behavior, aggressiveness, catatonic or disorganized behavior, possible suicide attempts.

Speech: Screaming or muteness, word salads (incomprehensible speech, severe loosening of associations).

Mood: Emotional turmoil.

Affect: Rapid shifts in affects. Inappropriate i.e, laughing at sad news, labile affect (abrupt fluctuations in affect).

Perception: Hallucinations.

Thought Process: Disorganized, loosening of associations.

Thought Content: Delusions, paranoid ideation.

Judgement: May be impaired.

Cognition: Disorientation, memory impairment, confusion.

Etiology/Predisposing Factors: Extreme stress; more likely to occur in individuals with borderline, histrionic, narcissistic, paranoid or schizotypal personalities.

Differential Diagnosis:

Brain injury or disease: Brain trauma, embolism, encephalitis, epilepsy (especially temporal lobe epilepsy), ischemia, tumor.

Systemic Disease: Hyperthyroidism, hypoglycemia, lupus erythematosus, multiple sclerosis, syphilis, vasculitis, vitamin deficiencies.

Psychiatric Disorders: Delirium, dementia, mood disorder with psychotic features, schizoaffective or schizophreniform disorder, psychogenic amnesia.

Treatment: Antipsychotics; may add benzodiazepines in conjunction with antipsychotics.

SELF TEST #6

1. All of the following are hypothesized causes of schizophrenia except:
   A) Genetic predisposition
   B) Excess dopamine activity
   C) Decreased dopamine activity
   D) High stress
2. All of the following are common symptoms of schizophrenia except:
   A) Blunted or flat affect
   B) Loosening of associations
   C) Aphasia
   D) Magical thinking
3. The most common hallucinations present in schizophrenia are:
   A) Gustatory
   B) Visual
   C) Olfactory
   D) Auditory
4. Your patient presents with delusions of persecution, aggressiveness and hallucinations related to a single paranoid theme. Which type of schizophrenia is your patient most likely suffering from:
   A) Disorganized
   B) Paranoid
   C) Catatonic
   D) Undifferentiated
5. Brief reactive psychosis is usually precipitated by:
   A) Extreme stress
   B) Antipsychotic medications
   C) Lack of stimulation
   D) Bipolar disorder

ANSWERS TO SELF TEST #6

1. The answer is C. **Decreased dopamine activity** is **not** thought to be a cause of schizophrenia.
2. The answer is C. **Aphasia** is not a common symptom of schizophrenia.
3. The answer is D. **Auditory** hallucinations are the most common hallucinations seen in schizophrenia.
4. The answer is B. Delusions of persecution, aggressiveness and hallucinations related to a single paranoid theme are characteristic of **paranoid** schizophrenia.

5. The answer is A. Brief reactive psychosis is usually precipitated by **extreme stress.**

ORGANIC MENTAL SYNDROMES

DELIRIUM

Definition: Altered state of consciousness induced by an underlying physical condition.

Behavior and psychomotor activity: Increase or decrease in psychomotor activity; reduced level of consciousness; tremors, sleep disturbances, fatigue, weakness, reduced frustration tolerance, distractibility, nightmares, amnesia for certain periods of time.

Speech: Incoherence, rambling.

Mood: Anxious, agitated, depressed mood; euphoria.

Affect: Labile (abrupt fluctuations of emotion).

Perception: Hallucinations (especially visual), illusions.

Thought process: Disorganized; impaired reasoning; loosening of associations (illogical shifting to unrelated topics).

Thought Content: Fear, paranoia, unsystemized delusions.

Cognition: Impairments in memory, inattentiveness, confusion, poor concentration; disorientation to time, place or person; inability to complete Digit Span test or Serial 7 test.

Etiology/Predisposing Factors:

Electrolyte imbalances, hypoglycemia, hypothyroidism, thyrotoxicosis, hypoxia, ketoacidosis, Addison's disease, Cushing's disease, pellagra, thiamine deficiency. meningitis, viral or AIDS encephalitis, pneumonia, septicemia, neoplasms, head trauma, transient ischemic attacks, epilepsy, hepatic encephalopathy, uremia, chronic obstructive pulmonary disease; heart or respiratory failure.

Drugs associated with delirium: Alcohol ingestion or withdrawal, amphetamines, anticonvulsants, antidepressants, antihistamines, antipsychotics, benztropine (Cogentin), clonidine, cocaine, corticosteroids, digoxin, disulfiram, hallucinogens, inhalants, levodopa, lidocaine, lithium, methyldopa, pentazocine, procainamide, beta-blockers.

Treatment: Treat underlying disorder. Benzodiazepines and antipsychotics may be used for extreme agitation or psychosis.

Differential Diagnosis: Psychotic disorders, anxiety, dementia, depression.

Studies to determine the etiology of delirium: Complete blood cell count, electrolytes, creatinine/BUN, glucose, liver panel, toxicology studies, calcium, phosphate, magnesium, VDRL, B12 and folate levels; thyroid function tests; EEG, ECG, CT/MRI.

DEMENTIA

Definition: Progressive mental deterioration and intellectual decline due to organic brain disease.

Appearance: Disheveled.

Behavior and psychomotor activity: Slowing of motor activity and thought; apraxia (loss of ability to carry out purposeful movements), hand tremors, unsteady gait.

Speech: Slow speech, perseveration (repetition of words or phrases), aphasia.

Affect: Labile (fluctuations of emotion).

Perception: Illusions, hallucinations (especially visual).

Thought Content: Delusions, paranoia, impaired judgment.

Cognition: Impaired abstract thinking, memory and cognitive impairments; disorientation, agnosia (loss of ability to recognize certain sensory stimuli).

Differential Diagnosis: Delirium, schizophrenia, major depression, Alzheimer's disease, Huntington's Chorea, Pick's disease, Jackob-Creutzfeldt's disease, meningitis, multiple sclerosis, multi-infarct dementia, Wilson's disease, hypothyroidism, hypoglycemia, B12 deficiency, hepatic encephalopathy, uremia, brain tumor, normal pressure hydrocephalus.

Drugs Associated with Dementia: Anticholinergics, solvent inhalants, metallic poisons, psychotropic agents, other drugs which affect CNS.

Treatment: Treat underlying disorder. Agitation may be treated with benzodiazepines or antipsychotics, depression may be treated with antidepressants.

ALZHEIMER'S DISEASE

Definition: A degenerative form of dementia characterized by slow onset with progressive deterioration in memory and cognitive function.

Appearance: Disheveled, focal neurologic signs.

Behavior and psychomotor activity: Personality changes, agitation, emotional outbursts, purposeless wandering, apraxia (loss of ability to carry out purposeful movements), hand tremors.

Speech: Slowed speech, perseveration (repetition of words or phrases), aphasia, anomia (inability to name objects). Disruption in sleep pattern.

Mood: Depression, euphoria.

Affect: Labile affect, agitation, anxiety, irritability.

Perception: Hallucinations or illusions.

Thought process: Impaired abstract thinking.

Thought Content: Delusions, impaired judgment.

Cognition: Progressive deterioration in memory. Agnosia (loss of ability to recognize certain sensory stimuli).

Etiology/Predisposing Factors: Advanced age, genetic predisposition, history of head trauma, Downs syndrome; neuropathologic lesions causing neurotransmitter deficiencies.

Differential Diagnosis: Delirium, multi-infarct dementia, major depression, Parkinson's disease, Huntington's disease, Pick's disease.

Treatment: Agitation and emotional liability may be treated with antipsychotics; depression may be treated with antidepressants.

MULTI-INFARCT DEMENTIA

Definition: Dementia with abrupt onset and a step-wise, fluctuating, progressively deteriorating course; affects certain functions, while leaving others intact.

Appearance: Possibly disheveled, focal neurologic signs.

Behavior and psychomotor activity: Apraxia (loss of ability to carry out purposeful movements), dysphagia, nocturnal confusion, somatic complaints.

Speech: Dysarthria, perseveration (repetition of words or phrases).

Mood: Depression, euphoria.

Affect: Labile affect, episodes of laughing or crying.

Perception: Visual hallucinations.

Thought process: Impaired abstract thinking, impaired judgement.

Cognition: Confusion, step-wise deterioration in functioning , impaired logical function, agnosia (loss of ability to recognize sensory stimuli).

Etiology/Predisposing Factors: Cerebrovascular disease.

Differential Diagnosis: Stroke, depression, Parkinson's disease, intracranial tumor.

Treatment: Reduce cholesterol intake; control of weight and blood pressure, cessation of smoking; anticoagulants may be of some benefit. Emotional liability and agitation may be treated with low doses of antipsychotics; depression may be treated with antidepressants.

DIFFERENTIATION OF DELIRIUM/DEMENTIA

	Delirium	Dementia
Onset:	Acute	Gradual
Course:	Fluctuating	Step-wise deterioration
Attention:	Inability to concentrate	May be able to concentrate
Duration:	Hours, days,	Months, weeks to years
Perception:	Frequent impairments	Less frequent Impairments
Sleep:	More disruption	Less disruption
EEG:	Diffuse slowing	Mild or normal
Prognosis:	Usually good	Poor .

ORGANIC DELUSIONAL SYNDROME

Definition: Delusions due to an organic brain disease.

Appearance: Unkept appearance, eccentric dress.

Behavior and psychomotor activity: Stereotyped behavior (repetition of certain activities); hyperactivity ; catatonic posturing (inappropriate strange postures); anxiety, psychomotor agitation or retardation.

Speech: Incoherence, rambling.

Mood: Normal to dysphoric.

Affect: Normal to flat.

Perception: Hallucinations (usually secondary to delusions).

Thought process: May be impaired.

Thought Content: Delusions (usually paranoid), impaired judgement; may act upon delusions.

Cognition: Minimal impairment.

Etiology/Predisposing Factors: Amphetamine or hallucinogen intoxication; cerebral lesions, temporal lobe epilepsy, multiple sclerosis, Wilson's disease, systemic lupus erythematosus, uremia.

Differential Diagnosis: Schizophrenia, organic mood disorder or delusional disorder.

Treatment: Treat underlying disorder, antipsychotics.

ORGANIC MOOD SYNDROME

Definition: Depressed, expansive or elevated mood due to an organic factor.

Behavior and psychomotor activity: Loss of interest in usual activities, suicidal ideation, impulsive or self destructive behavior are common; sleep disturbances, reduced libido, sleep impairments, weight loss.

Mood: Depressed, expansive or elevated mood.

Affect: Normal to flat.

Perception: Hallucinations may be present.

Thought Content: Delusions, pessimism, guilt.

Cognition: Mild impairment.

Etiology/Predisposing Factors: Stroke, viral encephalitis, endocrine and metabolic disorders, steroids, psychosis, hallucinogen intoxication; methyldopa.

Differential Diagnosis: Mood disorders, schizophrenia.

Treatment: Treat underlying disorder, treat depression with antidepressants.

ORGANIC PERSONALITY SYNDROME

Definition: Personality disturbance due to a specific organic disorder.

Behavior and psychomotor activity: Personality change, outbursts of anger, lack of interest in usual activities, apathy, indifference.

Mood: Depressed, anxious or irritable.

Affect: Labile affect.

Thought Content: Paranoid ideation; impaired social judgement, cognition.

Etiology/Predisposing Factors: Head trauma, intracranial tumors, temporal lobe epilepsy, Multiple sclerosis, Huntington's disease.

Differential Diagnosis: Delirium. dementia, mood disorder, schizophrenia.

Treatment: Treat underlying disorder.

ORGANIC HALLUCINOSIS

Definition: Hallucinations due to an organic disorder.

Mood: Anxious, fearful.

Affect: Normal to flat.

Perception: Auditory, visual and tactile hallucinations.

Thought Content: Ideas of reference (people, objects or events are believed to have a specific, unusual meaning). Fear of "losing one's mind", delusions.

Judgment: May be impaired and patient may act on hallucinations or delusions.
Etiology/Predisposing Factors: Alcohol abuse or withdrawal, hallucinogen intoxication, other medications, seizure disorder.
Differential Diagnosis: Schizophrenia, mood disorders, dementia, delirium, organic delusional syndrome, alcohol hallucinosis, seizure disorder, M.S.
Treatment: Treat underlying disorder.

SELF TEST #2

1. Signs of **delirium** include all of the following except:
   A) Reduced ability to maintain attention.
   B) Disorientation
   C) Disorganized thought process.
   D) Flat affect
2. All of the following are common in **dementia** except:
   A) Personality changes
   B) Aphasia
   C) Paranoia
   D) Neologisms
3. All of the following are signs of **Alzheimer's Disease** except:
   A) Progressive deterioration in mental functioning.
   B) Preservation
   C) Impairments abstract thinking.
   D) Ambivalence
4. In **organic delusional syndrome** all of the following are common except:
   A) Stereotyped behavior
   B) Incoherence
   C) Clanging
   D) Dysphoric mood

ANSWERS TO SELF TEST #2

1. The answer is D. **flat affect** is **not** common in delirium. labile affect is a common affect seen in delirium.
2. The answer is D. **Neologisms** are not common in dementia.
3. The answer is D. **Ambivalence** is not a sign of Alzheimer's Disease.
4. The answer is C. **Clanging** is not common in organic delusional syndrome.

ANXIETY DISORDERS AND STATES

GENERALIZED ANXIETY DISORDER

Definition: Excessive anxiety or worry for at least six months.

Appearance: Trembling, twitching, diaphoresis, clammy extremities.

Behavior and psychomotor activity: Restlessness, vigilance or scanning, irritability, difficulty concentrating; fatigability, insomnia, muscle tension, trouble swallowing, chills or hot flashes, cold sweats, dizziness, dyspnea, tremors, tachycardia, hypertension; GI upset; exaggerated startle response, sleep disturbances, frequent urination, headaches, hyperventilation, increased psychomotor behavior, multiple somatic complaints.

Mood: Excessive anxiety or worrying causing significant distress or dysfunction, feeling of being "keyed up" or "on edge". Mild depression is common.

Affect: Tense, anxious.

Thought Content: Fear of serious illness, sense of impending doom.

Etiology/Predisposing Factors: Psychological and biological factors; depression may be a predisposing factor.

Differential Diagnosis: Caffeine intoxication, nicotine and sedative withdrawal, hyperthyroidism, hypoglycemia, organic mental disorder, stimulant drugs, central nervous system depressant withdrawal. Cushing's syndrome, carcinoid syndrome, pheochromocytoma, hypercalcemia, porphyria, pulmonary embolism, mitral valve prolapse, hypertension, temporal lobe epilepsy, transient ischemic episode, Wilson's disease and Huntington's disease, Multiple Sclerosis.

Treatment: Psychotherapy, relaxation techniques, buspirone (Buspar), benzodiazepines, antidepressants.

PANIC DISORDER

Definition: Unexpected attacks of anxiety.

Appearance: Shaking, trembling, diaphoresis.

Behavior and psychomotor activity: Restlessness, pacing, faintness, chills, hot flashes, tachycardia, choking sensations, dyspnea, nausea, abdominal distress, sleep disturbances, diaphoresis, GI upset, paresthesias, tremors.

Perception: Depersonalization, derealization.

Mood: Depression and/or intense anxiety.

Thought Content: Confusion, fear of dying or "going crazy", sense of impending doom. Patient may believe he or she has a medical problem.

Etiology/Predisposing Factors: Separation anxiety disorder in childhood; mitral valve prolapse. Biologic and genetic factors, major depression; alcoholism may predispose.

Differential Diagnosis: Hypoglycemia, hyperthyroidism, pheochromocytoma, psychoactive substance intoxication or withdrawal, generalized anxiety disorder, phobia, caffeine intoxication; nicotine and sedative withdrawal, organic mental disorder; stimulant drugs; central nervous system depressant withdrawal. Cushing's syndrome, carcinoid syndrome, hypercalcemia, porphyria, hypertension, temporal lobe epilepsy, transient ischemic episode, Wilson's and Huntington's disease, multiple sclerosis.

Treatment: Psychotherapy, behavior modification, relaxation techniques; tricyclic antidepressants, fluoxetine (Prozac), MAO inhibitors; benzodiazepines (especially alprazolam), beta blockers.

PANIC DISORDER WITH AGORAPHOBIA

Definition: Unexpected attacks of anxiety, and a fear and avoidance of crowded, open or unfamiliar places.

Appearance: Shaking, trembling.

Behavior and psychomotor activity: Apprehension, restlessness, pacing, diaphoresis, dizziness, chills, hot flashes, tachycardia, choking sensations, dyspnea, nausea or abdominal distress, faintness, sleep disturbances, GI upset, paresthesias.

Mood: Depression and anxiety are common.

Perception: Depersonalization (feeling of being outside of oneself), derealization (feelings of unrealness involving the outer environment).

Thought Content: Fear of not being able to escape from feared place; fear of being embarrassed or "going crazy".

Etiology/Predisposing Factors: Separation anxiety disorder in childhood, mitral valve prolapse.

Differential Diagnosis: Hypoglycemia, hyperthyroidism, pheochromocytoma, psychoactive substance intoxication or withdrawal; generalized anxiety disorder, simple or social phobia, caffeine intoxication, nicotine and sedative withdrawal, organic mental disorder, stimulant drugs, central nervous system depressant withdrawal. Cushing's syndrome, carcinoid syndrome, hypercalcemia, porphyria, hypertension, temporal lobe epilepsy, transient ischemic episode.

Treatment: Psychotherapy, behavior modification, relaxation techniques, tricyclic antidepressants, fluoxetine (Prozac), MAO inhibitors, benzodiazepines, beta blockers.

POST TRAUMATIC STRESS DISORDER

Definition: Following a traumatic event repeatedly reexperiencing the event. (military combat, rape, natural disaster).

Behavior and psychomotor activity: Reexperiencing traumatic event through dreams, flashbacks and memories. Depressed responsiveness to environment; feeling of being detached from others, avoidance of activities or stimuli associated with traumatic event; loss of interest in usual activities, aggressiveness; substance abuse, sleep disorders, difficulty concentrating, outbursts of anger, nightmares.

Mood: Depression is common.

Affect: Restricted affect, anxiety, irritability.

Perception: Illusions pertaining to the trauma.

Thought Content: Intrusive thoughts or images of the traumatic event.

Etiology/Predisposing Factors: Experiencing of an extremely traumatic event

Differential Diagnosis: Depression, bipolar disorder, anxiety, adjustment disorder, schizophrenia, some organic mental disorders.

Treatment: Psychotherapy, group therapy, tricyclic antidepressants, carbamazepine, propranolol (Inderal).

OBSESSIVE COMPULSIVE DISORDER

Definition: Compulsions (stereotyped behavior performed to alleviate anxiety in response to an obsession) i.e., hand washing in response to feeling one has been contaminated. The compulsions are time consuming and interfere with activities, and are undesired and uncontrollable; patients may hide their compulsions from others.

Appearance: Normal

Speech: Normal

Mood: Anxiety and depression are common.

Thought Content: Intrusive thoughts, impulses or images such as thoughts of harming another person or being contaminated.

Judgement: The patient recognizes that his thoughts and behavior are illogical.

Etiology/Predisposing Factors: Psychological factors, serotonin functions, family history of obsessive compulsive disorder.

Differential Diagnosis: Depression, phobic disorder, schizophrenia, Tourette's syndrome, phobia.

Treatment: Psychotherapy, behavioral modification, antidepressants; clomipramine, fluoxetine, sertraline.

MEDICAL CONDITIONS WITH PSYCHIATRIC SYMPTOMS

Addison's Disease: Apathy, depression, fatigue, weakness.
Cushing's Syndrome: Depression, euphoria, anxiety, somatic delusions.
Hyperthyroidism: Anxiety, hyperactivity, irritability, impulsiveness, restlessness, rapid pressured speech, weight loss, psychosis.
Hypothyroidism: Depression, apathy, fatigue, withdrawal.
Hyperparathyroidism: Depression, anxiety, anorexia, fatigue, confusion, delusions, hallucinations.
Acute intermittent porphyria: Labile affect, anxiety, depression, irritability, hallucinations and delusions, psychosis.
Huntington's Chorea: Schizophrenia like psychosis, anxiety, personality changes.
Hyper/Hyponatremia Depression, anxiety.
Mitral Valve Prolapse: Anxiety, panic attacks.
Pellagra: Insomnia, delusions, dementia, depression.
Systemic Lupus Erythematosus: Depression, toxic psychosis, delirium.
Intracranial Tumors: Anxiety, depression, personality change; impaired memory, judgement, cognition.
Pernicious Anemia: Depression, fatigue, dementia.
Temporal Lobe Epilepsy: Illusions, inappropriate fear or anger; time distortion, deja vu (feeling of familiarity with surroundings), depression, hallucinations, dissociative states, paranoia, delusional syndromes, psychosis, personality changes.
Encephalitis: Personality change, labile affect, confusion, delirium.
Multiple Sclerosis: Depression, anxiety, delirium, dementia.

MEDICATIONS ASSOCIATED WITH PSYCHIATRIC SYMPTOMS

Phenobarbital: Irritability, sedation, confusion.
Anticholinergics: Psychosis, organic brain syndrome.
Antihypertensives: Depression, delirium.
Cimetidine: Toxic psychosis, depression, mania.
L-Dopa: Anxiety, agitation, delirium, depression, psychosis.
Oral Contraceptives: Depression, anxiety.

Digitalis: Delirium, depression, anxiety.

Quinidine: Delirium.

Procainamide: Depression, delusions, hallucinations.

Disopyramide: Hallucinations, panic, depression.

Lidocaine: Delirium.

Phenytoin: Depression, irritability, hallucinations.

Amantadine: Insomnia, nightmares, delirium, confusion, acute mania.

Bromocriptine: Paranoia, hallucinations, acute mania.

Disulfiram: Depression, paranoia, delirium.

SUBSTANCE USE DISORDERS

ALCOHOLISM

Definition: Physiologic dependence, tolerance, inability to abstain from consumption, and withdrawal symptoms upon continuation.

Signs/Symptoms of Intoxication: Slurred speech, ataxia, impaired judgement, disinhibition, mood disturbances, paranoia, hypothermia, tachycardia, dilated pupils, nystagmus, coma.

Signs/Symptoms of Withdrawal: Tremors, hallucinations, nausea, vomiting, diarrhea, headaches, weakness, fever; impaired memory, judgment and concentration; sleep disturbances, anxiety, depression, hypertension, irritability, tachycardia, convulsions.

Etiology/Predisposing Factors: Genetic predisposition and psychological factors may contribute.

Treatment of Intoxication: Unconscious patient: protect against Wernicke's encephalopathy with thiamine; treat excess intracranial pressure, hypoglycemia, maintain airway.

Conscious patient: treat violent or agitated patients with restraints or sedation. Benzodiazepines for sedation, vitamin supplements, low dose haloperidol for psychosis.

Treatment of Addiction: Detoxification, psychotherapy, group therapy (Alcoholics Anonymous), disulfiram (Antabuse)

Treatment of Withdrawal: Treat dehydration with fluids, diazepam, lorazepam or phenobarbital for withdrawal seizures. Treat tremors with benzodiazepines; thiamine 100 mg IM per day for three days to prevent Wernicke's encephalopathy. Treat delirium with benzodiazepines, antipsychotics in severe cases.

OPIATE NARCOTIC ABUSE

Opiate Drugs: Codeine, hydrocodone, hydromorphone (Dilaudid), methadone, morphine, oxycodone (Percodan), oxymorphone (Numorphan), propoxyphene (Darvon).

Signs/Symptoms of Intoxication: Euphoria or dysphoria, lethargy, nausea, vomiting, analgesia, slurred speech, respiratory depression, miosis, hypotension, hypoactive reflexes, hypothermia, bradycardia, seizures.

Signs/Symptoms of Addiction: Inability to abstain from consumption, tolerance; withdrawal symptoms upon discontinuation, anxiety, depression.

Signs/Symptoms of Withdrawal: Drug craving, anxiety, irritability, sweating, yawning, muscle twitching or cramping; insomnia, rhinorrhea, diaphoresis, pupillary dilation, hot or cold flashes; diarrhea, nausea, vomiting, restlessness, hypertension, tachycardia.

Treatment of Intoxication: Supportive measures, naloxone.

Treatment of Withdrawal: Detoxification, benzodiazepines; psychotherapy, group therapy; methadone, clonidine, naltrexone.

MARIJUANA ABUSE

Signs/Symptoms of Intoxication: Euphoria, anxiety; behavioral and personality changes, sensation that time has slowed down; increased appetite; suggestibility, dry mouth, conjunctival injection, panic attacks, tachycardia, impaired motor performance, delusional syndrome, lethargy, depression, lack of motivation.

Signs/Symptoms of Addiction: Inability to abstain from consumption, tolerance.

Signs/ Symptoms of Withdrawal: Irritability, insomnia, sweating.

Treatment of Intoxication: Treat panic with benzodiazepines.

Treatment of Addiction: Psychotherapy, behavioral modification, group therapy.

HALLUCINOGENS

Hallucinogens of Abuse: Lysergic acid diethylamide (LSD), mescaline, psilocybin (magic mushrooms), 2,5-dimethoxy-4-methylamphetamine (STP), Ketamine MDMA (Ecstasy).

Signs/Symptoms of Intoxication: Hyperreflexia, diaphoresis, mydriasis, blurred vision, ataxia, hypertension, tachycardia, tremor, hyperthermia, illusions, hallucinations, depersonalization, anxiety, sense of increased insight; mystical experiences, paranoia, psychosis.

Signs/Symptoms of Addiction: Hallucinogens do not produce tolerance.

Treatment of Intoxication: Treat psychotic symptoms and flashbacks with antipsychotics; Treat delirium with haloperidol, dark quiet room. Treat anxiety and restlessness with diazepam.

PHENCYCLIDINE (PCP) ABUSE

Signs/Symptoms of Intoxication: Violent behavior, belligerence, euphoria, hyperactivity, hypersensitivity to stimuli, anxiety, confusion, perceptual distortions, floating sensations, paranoia, psychosis, catatonia, ataxia, incoordination, diaphoresis, tachycardia, dysarthria, lack of sensitivity to pain, nystagmus, fever, clonic jerking, intracranial hemorrhage, seizures, coma, death.
Signs/Symptoms of Addiction: PCP does not produce tolerance.
Signs/Symptoms of Withdrawal: Occasional depression.
Treatment of Intoxication: Benzodiazepines, quiet room, haloperidol for violence.

PERSONALITY DISORDERS

BORDERLINE PERSONALITY DISORDER

Definition: A personality disorder characterized by impulsive or unpredictable behavior, and inability to control temper.
Behavior: Manipulative suicidal gestures; lack of satisfaction, anger, hostile behavior; dependent relationships alternating with devaluation, emptiness or boredom, unstable self image, difficulty being alone; volatile interpersonal relationships; possible substance abuse, engagement in impulsive acts; poor social adaptation.
Mood: Depression and dysphoria are common.
Affect: Labile affect, anxiety, irritability.
Thought Content: Cognitive distortions, fears of being abandoned; pessimism and apathy; Use of defense mechanisms such as acting out, denial, dissociation and splitting.
Etiology/Predisposing Factors: Experiential and psychological factors.
Differential Diagnosis: Identity disorder, depression, organic disorders (temporal lobe epilepsy, substance abuse, delirium), psychotic disorders, histrionic, antisocial and narcissistic personality disorders.
Treatment: Psychotherapy, behavior modification, antidepressants, lithium and antipsychotics are sometimes used.

HISTRIONIC PERSONALITY DISORDER

Definition: A personality disorder characterized by immature, seductive or manipulative behavior.

Behavior: Egocentricity; excessive concern with appearance, rejection of others, attention seeking behavior, fickleness, exhibitionism, aggression.

Appearance: Seductive, exhibitionistic dress and provocative behavior.

Mood: Emotionality

Speech: Impressionistic or overgeneralized, excessive use of superlatives.

Affect: Labile, irritable, exaggeration of emotional expression.

Thought Content: Romantic fantasizing is common; raving for attention and excitement, shallowness, low frustration tolerance, constant need for excessive praise and approval; use of certain defense mechanisms such as acting out, denial, dissociation and splitting.

Etiology/Predisposing Factors: Experiential and psychological causes.

Differential Diagnosis: Narcissistic personality disorder, borderline personality disorder, antisocial personality disorder.

Treatment: Psychotherapy, behavior modification.

OBSESSIVE COMPULSIVE PERSONALITY DISORDER

Definition: A personality disorder characterized by perfectionism, obstinacy (inflexibility), preoccupation with order and detail (rules and lists).

Behavior: Need to be in complete control, excessive self consciousness, perseverance; obsessions related to everyday problems, lack of participation in leisure activities, dullness, lack of provocativeness, indecisiveness, parsimony (excessive frugality).

Appearance: Meticulous grooming and dress.

Attitude: Extreme seriousness.

Speech: Detailed responses to questions.

Mood: Anxiety and depression are common.

Affect: Constricted affect (inability to express warmth or tenderness).

Thought Content: Defense mechanisms include displacement, isolation, intellectualization, reaction formation and undoing.

Etiology/Predisposing Factors: Experiential, genetic and psychological factors.

Differential Diagnosis: Obsessive compulsive disorder, schizoid personality disorder.

Treatment: Psychotherapy, behavioral modification, group therapy.

NARCISSISTIC PERSONALITY DISORDER

Definition: A personality disorder characterized by interpersonal exploitation, constant seeking of attention and admiration; preoccupation with physical appearance of self and others.

Behavior: Inappropriate feelings of worthlessness and inferiority.

Attitude: Grandiosity.

Mood Depressed mood is common.

Thought Content: Hypersensitivity to criticism; lack of empathy, envious feelings, unstable self-esteem; belief that one is entitled to special favors without reciprocating, preoccupation with fantasies (ideal love, unlimited success).

Etiology/Predisposing Factors Experiential and psychological factors

Differential Diagnosis: Borderline, antisocial or histrionic personality disorders.

Treatment: Psychotherapy, behavior modification, antidepressants, lithium.

SCHIZOID PERSONALITY DISORDER

Definition: A personality disorder characterized by social isolation, inability to form close relationships, lack of libido, indifference to praise or criticism; indecisiveness, egocentric behavior; coldness, aloofness. Indifference to the opinions, needs, feelings of others.

Appearance: Patient appears uncomfortable and lacks eye contact.

Affect: Restricted affect, inability to express anger.

Thought Process: Brief answers to questions are common, forgetfulness.

Thought Content: Excessive fantasizing. Use of certain defense mechanisms such as projection and fantasy.

Etiology/Predisposing Factors: Genetic, biological, experiential and psychological factors.

Differential Diagnosis: Avoidant or schizotypal personality disorders.

Treatment: Group therapy, psychotherapy.

SCHIZOTYPAL PERSONALITY DISORDER

Definition: A personality disorder characterized by peculiarities of thought and behavior similar to those of schizophrenia.

Appearance: Dress may be peculiar, lack of facial expression.

Behavior and Psychomotor Activity: Social isolation.

Speech: Unclear speech, usually requires interpretation.

Mood: Anxiety and depression are common.

Affect: Flat, restricted, inappropriate.

Perception: Illusions, depersonalization.

Thought Process: Disordered, talks to self.

Content of Thought: Odd or paranoid ideation, magical thinking, ideas of reference (persons or objects take on special meaning), suspiciousness, Use of projection and fantasy.

Etiology/Predisposing Factors: Biological, experiential or psychological factors.

Differential Diagnosis: Borderline, schizoid, avoidant personality disorder; early schizophrenia.

Treatment: Group therapy, psychotherapy, low doses of antipsychotics.

AVOIDANT PERSONALITY DISORDER

Definition: Desire to please and be accepted, desire for but avoidance of relationships due to fear of being hurt; avoidance and fear of social activity.

Appearance: Anxious.

Attitude: Ingratiating

Behavior and Psychomotor Activity: Hypersensitivity to rejection, lack of assertiveness, fragile self-esteem, shyness, over-sensitivity; extreme anxiety in social situations; misinterpretation of remarks as being critical or derogatory.

Mood: Anxious and depressed mood.

Thought Content: Use of defense mechanisms such as isolation and passive aggression.

Etiology/Predisposing Factors: Experiential and psychological causes.

Differential Diagnosis: Schizoid personality disorder, social phobia, panic disorder, panic disorder with agoraphobia.

Treatment: Psychotherapy, group therapy, behavioral modification, assertiveness training. Possible improvement with MAO inhibitors, beta blockers.

PARANOID PERSONALITY DISORDER

Definition: Unwarranted suspiciousness of others; lack of interest in other people.

Behavior: Inability to trust others; refusal to acknowledge responsibility for the ones feelings; intolerance for persons with illnesses or defects. Blaming others for one's feelings; unwarranted accusing of partner of infidelity, moralistic attitude; litigious behavior, fear of close relationships.

Appearance: Tenseness, scanning of environment; may behave in an overly business like manner.

Speech: Logical, formal.

Mood: Easily provoked to anger.

Affect: Restricted

Perception: Illusions are common.

Thought Content: Ideas of reference, projection, prejudice. Use of defense mechanisms such as fantasy and projection.

Judgement: May be impaired.

Etiology/Predisposing Factors: Experiential, psychological and organic factors.

Differential Diagnosis: Paranoid schizophrenia, delusional disorder, psychoactive substance abuse.

Treatment: Psychotherapy, behavior modification, low dose antipsychotics.

ANTISOCIAL PERSONALITY DISORDER/SOCIOPATHY

Definition: A personality disorder characterized by lack of conscience, egocentricity, inability to control impulses; violating the rights of others.

Behavior: Substance abuse, promiscuity (inability to be faithful to partner); pathological lying, stealing, recklessness, irritability, aggressiveness, superficial charm, multiple unwanted pregnancies; irresponsible behavior regarding children, inability to sustain or retain employment; defaults on loans, suicide threats, somatic complaints, use of aliases.

Mood: Depression, anxiety are common but may be denied.

Affect: Normal

Thought Content: Use of defense mechanisms such as acting out, denial, dissociation and splitting.

Etiology/Predisposing Factors: Possibly early childhood experiences of a negative nature; family history of alcoholism, genetic or biological factors.

Differential Diagnosis: Conduct disorder, alcoholism, substance abuse, antisocial behavior due to another cause, borderline or histrionic personality disorder.

Treatment: Psychotherapy, group therapy.

DEPENDENT PERSONALITY DISORDER

Definition: A personality disorder characterized by passiveness, lack of initiative, extreme sensitivity to criticism, low self esteem

Behavior: Difficulty expressing aggressive or sexual feelings, helplessness, pessimism, going to extreme lengths to be accepted; experiences extreme difficulty when relationships end. Tends to agree with others point of view to avoid rejection; inability to make decisions without excessive advice or allowing other to make decisions and reliance on others to make decisions; intolerance to being alone, lack of self reliance, fear of abandonment or rejection.

Etiology/Predisposing Factors: Experiential and psychological factors.

Differential Diagnosis: Passive-aggressive and avoidant personality disorder, schizophrenia.

Treatment: Psychotherapy, behavior modification, assertiveness training.

PASSIVE AGGRESSIVE PERSONALITY DISORDER

Definition: Sulking, negativism (refusal to cooperate, often doing the exact opposite of what is requested), indirect expression of anger through procrastination and makes excuses for delays;

Behavior: Refusal to perform adequately in work or social situations; "forgetting" obligations, stubbornness, lack of assertiveness; resentment and manipulation of others; finds excessive fault in others.

Thought Content: Use of defense mechanisms such as denial, rationalization, or isolation, blames others for problems; finds excessive fault in others, thinks he has been treated unjustly, hypochondriacal concerns.

Etiology/Predisposing Factors: Experiential or psychological factors.

Differential Diagnosis: Borderline and dependent personality disorder, depression.

Treatment: Psychotherapy, cognitive therapy, behavior modification.

SADISTIC PERSONALITY DISORDER

Definition: A personality disorder characterized by cruel and aggressive behavior; humiliation, intimidation and domination of others.

Behavior: Violent and enjoys causing suffering; harshly punishes people under his control.

Etiology/Predisposing Factors: Child abuse may predispose to this disorder.

Differential Diagnosis: Antisocial personality disorder.

Treatment: Psychotherapy, behavior modification.

SELF TEST #8

1. Fears of being abandoned, chronic emptiness or boredom, manipulative suicidal gestures, self destructive behavior, and unstable self image are symptoms of which of the following personality disorders:

A) Histrionic
B) Borderline
C) Narcissistic
D) Avoidant

2. Grandiosity, preoccupation with fantasies, hypersensitivity to criticism, lack of empathy, need for admiration, are characteristics of what personality disorder:
A) Schizoid
B) Narcissistic
C) Histrionic
D) Sadistic

3. Schizoid personality disorder is characterized by all of the following except:
A) Social isolation
B) Loss of libido
C) Aloofness
D) Seductiveness

4. Suspiciousness, ideas of reference, jealousness and paranoia are all characteristics of what personality disorder:
A) Paranoid
B) Antisocial
C) Borderline
D) Schizoid

5. Passiveness, low self esteem, reliance on others to make decisions and fear of rejection are characteristic of what personality disorder:
A) Schizoid
B) Passive/aggressive
C) Dependent
D) Obsessive/compulsive

ANSWERS TO SELF TEST #8

1. The answer is B. These are all common symptoms of **borderline personality disorder**.
2. The answer is B. These are characteristics of **narcissistic personality disorder**.
3. The answer is D. **Seductiveness** is not a common characteristic of schizoid personality disorder.
4. The answer is A. Suspiciousness, ideas of reference, jealousness,and paranoia are all common characteristics of **paranoid personality disorder**.
5.The answer is C. Reliance on others to make decisions and fear of rejection are

characteristics of **dependent personality disorder.**

SOMATOFORM DISORDERS

CONVERSION DISORDER

Definition: Conversion of a psychological conflict or stress into a deficit of physical functioning. The patient is not in control of symptoms.

Signs/Symptoms: Sudden onset after a stressful event. Paralysis, blindness, seizures, paresthesias, anesthesia, ataxia, aphonia (loss of speech), loss of sensation, fainting, vomiting, deafness, weakness, tremors.

Etiology/Predisposing Factors: Psychological factors. More common in persons with histrionic or hysterical personalities.

Differential Diagnosis: Multiple sclerosis, neurological disorder, malingering, somatization disorder, factitious disorder.

Treatment: Rule out physical causes; psychotherapy, hypnosis or amobarbital interview. Benzodiazepines for anxiety.

SOMATIZATION DISORDER (BRIQUET'S SYNDROME, HYSTERIA)

Definition: Multiple physical complaints with no evidence of physical illness.

Signs/Symptoms: Usually complaints are presented in a dramatic way, long detailed medical history; symptoms include pain in extremities, joints, back; pelvic pain, shortness of breath, chest pain, palpitations, dizziness, nausea, vomiting, abdominal pain, diarrhea, food intolerance, difficulty swallowing; psychosexual symptoms, menstrual pain, amnesia, paralysis, blindness, seizures, paresthesias, anesthesia, ataxia, aphonia (loss of speech), akinesia, dyskinesia, loss of sensation, fainting, vomiting, deafness, weakness, tunnel vision, tremors. preoccupation with one's self, dependant and seductive tendencies.

Associated Features: Depression, anxiety, alcohol and drug abuse, interpersonal difficulties, manipulative behavior.

Etiology/Predisposing Factors: Theories include genetic components, repressed impulses. Increased incidence in persons with first-degree male relatives with alcoholism or sociopathy, or female relatives with somatization disorder.

Differential Diagnosis: Physical illnesses such as multiple sclerosis, hyperparathyroidism, porphyria, temporal lobe epilepsy, systemic lupus erythematosus, schizophrenia, malingering.

Treatment: Psychotherapy, avoidance of unnecessary procedures and medications.

SOMATOFORM PAIN DISORDER

Definition: Experiencing pain for which no physical cause can be found or experiencing pain out of proportion to an existing physical factor.

Signs/Symptoms: Obsession with pain; extensive medical/surgical history, depression may be present.

Etiology/Predisposing Factors: Working at an early age, need to play the sick role. Possible genetic components; altered regulation of endorphins or monoamine neurotransmitters.

Differential Diagnosis: Pain with organic origin, conversion disorder, somatoform disorder, malingering, hypochondriasis, depression.

Treatment: Psychotherapy, behavioral modification, hypnosis, biofeedback, antidepressants.

BODY DYSMORPHIC DISORDER

Definition: Imagined defect in appearance (i.e., nose, wrinkles, breasts).

Signs/Symptoms: Obsession with imagined defect, depression, insomnia, defect may cause anxiety in social situations, perfectionistic traits, consultation with specialists in the area of imagined defect.

Etiology/Predisposing Factors: Psychological factors.

Differential Diagnosis: Delusional disorder, anorexia nervosa, obsessive compulsive disorder.

Treatment: Psychotherapy, tricyclic antidepressants (clomipramine), pimozide (Orap) is sometimes used.

HYPOCHONDRIASIS

Definition: Excessive worry or belief that one is suffering from a physical illness in spite of lack of medical evidence.

Signs/Symptoms: Anxiety, depression; "doctor shopping", vague complaints or symptoms, preoccupation with health and body functions, symptoms disproportionate to disease; complaints involving multiple organ systems (most commonly GI and cardiovascular complaints), fear of disease, extensive medical history; demanding or hostile behavior, anxiety, depression.

Etiology/Predisposing Factors: Psychological factors, medical treatment or hospitalization during childhood.

Differential Diagnosis: Physical illness, somatization disorder, depression, panic disorder, generalized anxiety disorder, delusional disorder.

Treatment: Psychotherapy, behavioral modifications; treat depression and anxiety.

EATING DISORDERS

ANOREXIA NERVOSA

Definition: An eating disorder characterized by excessive fear of gaining weight; loss of 15% body weight or more; amenorrhea; distorted body image.

Signs/Symptoms: Preoccupation with food; excessive exercising, yellow skin (carotinemia); abuse of diuretics, laxatives, cathartics; depression, anxiety, hypothermia, nutritional depletion.

Associated Features: Depression, GI disturbances, cold intolerance, insomnia, fatigue, decreased libido; compulsive behavior, denial of illness.

Medical Complications: Anemia, electrolyte imbalances, abdominal pain; bradycardia, arrhythmias, hypothermia, hypotension; increased serum carotene, diabetes insipidus, renal calculi, elevated liver enzymes, leukopenia, thrombocytopenia.

Etiology/Predisposing Factors: Stressful parent-child relations; perfectionist traits. Hysterical, obsessive-compulsive or schizoid personality disorders.

Differential Diagnosis: Bulimia nervosa, chronic illness, superior mesenteric artery syndrome, hysterical refusal to eat, schizophrenia, Addison's Disease, hyper or hypothyroidism, intracranial tumor, physiologic thin structure.

Treatment: Psychotherapy, behavior modification, nutritional counseling; hospitalization, supervised feedings; cyproheptadine to stimulate appetite, antidepressants for associated depression.

BULIMIA

Definition: An eating disorder characterized by binge eating (consuming large amounts of food in one sitting), self-induced vomiting.

Signs/Symptoms: Weight may be normal; fasting, dieting; abuse of diuretics or laxative; depression, excessive concern with weight and body proportions; fluctuations in weight; feeling out of control of eating habits, preoccupation with food.

Associated Features: Depression, substance abuse, stealing food.

Complications: Esophageal tears, esophagitis, metabolic abnormalities, loss of enamel and decalcification of teeth; anemia, menstrual irregularities, gastric rupture, parotid gland swelling, hypokalemia, elevated serum amylase.
Differential Diagnosis: Anorexia, Kleine-Levin Syndrome, seizure disorder, depression, intracranial tumor, mood disorder, borderline personality disorder.
Treatment: Psychotherapy, hospitalization, nutritional counseling; medical stabilization, antidepressants.

OTHER DISORDERS

INSOMNIA

Definition: Inability to initiate or maintain sleep causing impairment in functioning.
Etiology/Predisposing Factors: Stress, depression, manic disorder, anxiety, physical illness, stimulants, caffeine, alcohol, daytime napping, nightmares, propranolol; antidepressants, reserpine; withdrawal from sedatives or hypnotics.
Treatment: Psychotherapy, relaxation techniques, exercise.

Flurazepam (Dalmane) 15-30 mg PO qhs.
Lorazepam (Ativan) 0.5-2 mg PO qhs.
Oxazepam (Serax) 15-30 mg PO qhs.
Temazepam (Restoril) 15-30 mg PO qhs.
Triazolam (Halcion) 0.125-0.25 mg PO qhs.

MULTIPLE PERSONALITY DISORDER

Definition: The presence of one or more personalities in the single patient.
Signs/Symptoms: The person may lose track of time while another personality is in control and each personality has its own patterns of behavior, attitudes, beliefs, memories and relationships. Transition from one personality to another is usually sudden, the patient may or may not be aware that the other personalities exist; depression and anxiety are common.
Etiology/Predisposing Factors: Severe emotional or physical abuse in childhood.
Differential Diagnosis: Schizophrenia, psychogenic fugue or amnesia, temporal lobe epilepsy, somnambulism, borderline personality disorder.
Treatment: Psychotherapy, hypnotherapy, group therapy.

FACTITIOUS DISORDER WITH PSYCHOLOGICAL SYMPTOMS

Definition: Patient invents symptoms of a psychological disorder.
Signs/Symptoms: Exhibition of symptoms only when aware of being observed, constant exhibiting of new symptoms unrelated to previous conditions, lack of response to therapeutic measures, exhibiting of symptoms observed in other patients, exaggeration of, or invention of new symptoms upon discharge from the hospital.
Etiology/Predisposing Factors: Psychological factors, desire to be considered ill.
Differential Diagnosis: Psychotic disorders, antisocial personality disorder, malingering, dementia.
Treatment: Psychotherapy, behavioral modification.

FACTITIOUS DISORDER WITH PHYSICAL SYMPTOMS

Definition: Patient invents symptoms of a physical disorder.
Signs/Symptoms: Obtaining treatment from multiple hospitals or doctors, desire to undergo invasive procedures; lack of visitors while in hospital, self-inflicted injury; pathological lying, insistence on medication, extensive medical history, surgical scarring (gridiron abdomen), lack of concern when undergoing surgical procedures; evasiveness, manipulation of hospital staff, familiarity with hospital procedures and medical terminology; new complaints as suspected illnesses are ruled out, interference with diagnostic procedures, angry, hostile, disruptive behavior in the hospital and substance abuse are common.
Etiology/Predisposing Factors: Psychological factors, extensive medical treatment or hospitalization in childhood, abuse as a child.
Differential Diagnosis: True physical disorder, malingering, somatoform disorder, hypochondriasis.
Treatment Psychotherapy, prevention of unnecessary procedures.

DELUSIONAL DISORDERS

Definition: Disorder in which the patient has firm beliefs that have no factual basis.
Erotomania: False belief that another person is in love with the patient.
Grandiose: Inflated self worth or feeling that one has a special relationship with a prominent figure.
Jealous: Belief that a partner has been unfaithful.

Persecutory: Belief that one is being persecuted, spied on or in danger of being harmed by others.

Somatic: False belief that one has a defect or illness. Patient may consult with specialist in the area of the imagined defect.

Differential Diagnosis: Conditions associated with delusions include: Addison's disease, Cushing's syndrome, brain tumor, cerebrovascular disease, delirium, dementia, Multiple sclerosis, subdural hematoma, temporal lobe epilepsy, certain metabolic and endocrine disorders, AIDS, syphilis, encephalitis. Medications associated with delusions include: alcohol withdrawal, amphetamines, anticholinergics, barbiturates, bromocriptine, bupropion, cimetidine, cocaine, cortisone, disulfiram, hallucinogens, marijuana, methyldopa.

Treatment: Psychotherapy, antipsychotics, primozide (Orap).

BASIC PSYCHOLOGY

Types of Therapy

Supportive Therapy: The main goal in supportive therapy is to encourage the patient to become more functional by helping him to assess the situation and help make appropriate changes. The therapist listens to the patient and provides empathy, reassurance, and suggestions.

Cognitive Therapy: Therapists work with patients on correcting dysfunctional patterns of thinking. Therapists use various verbal procedures and behavioral modification techniques to help the patient correct faulty thought patterns.

Psychoanalytic Psychotherapy: The goal is to make major changes in the personality and maladaptive defense mechanisms of the patient by working through unconscious conflicts. Psychoanalytic psychotherapy is usually indicated in patients with obsessive compulsive disorders, symptomatic anxiety, and other neuroses. Patients who are highly motivated, able to form relationships, and have a capacity for insight are the best candidates.

Behavior Therapy: The goal of behavior therapy is to alter involuntary learned maladaptive behavior patterns. Techniques used include: Aversion (when undesired behavior occurs, punishment results i.e. spanking), implosion (the patient is instructed to imagine being exposed to the situation he fears or is anxious about), operant conditioning (use of positive or negative reinforcement), systemic desensitization (the patient is taken to the feared situation and gradually exposed to increasing degrees).

Group Therapy: Group therapy is a form of treatment where patients with disorders or problems are placed in a group with a trained therapist. The therapist uses group interactions to facilitate change.

Family Therapy: In family therapy the therapist meets with the family and each member individually. Therapists work on correcting dysfunctional communication skills and other specific problems.

Marital Therapy: The therapist works with the couple on communication, interacting and on resolving conflict

DEFENSE MECHANISMS:

Acting out: Impulsive behavior without concern for the effect actions will have.

Controlling: Minimizing anxiety by attempting to manipulate or control objects in ones environment.

Denial: Refusal to acknowledge some painful aspect of reality.

Devaluation: Negative qualities of ones self are attributed to others.

Displacement: Shifting of a feeling about an object or person onto another less threatening object.

Distortion: Reshaping of reality (hallucinations, delusions).

Externalization: Elements of personality are seen in external objects or people.

Idealization: Attributing excessive positive qualities to others or self.

Intellectualization: Use of intellectual thinking to avoid expression or experience.

Isolation: Separation of an idea from its affect (feelings about an idea are kept from consciousness).

Projection: Attributing of ones own feelings or thoughts to another person.

Rationalization: Justifying beliefs, attitudes or behavior through logical explanations.

Reaction formation: Substituting opposite feelings for actual feelings.

Repression: Keeping ideas, memories or feelings out of consciousness.

Schizoid/Autistic fantasy: Retreating into daydreaming and fantasizing, which substitutes for normal activities or relationships.

Sexualization: Giving sexual significance to objects or people in order to minimize anxiety.

Somatization: Conversion of psychological factors into physical symptoms.

Splitting: Dividing of self, others, or objects into all good or all bad categories often shifting from one extreme to another.

Suppression: Avoidance of thoughts of disturbing conflicts, feelings or experie-nces.

THERAPEUTIC AGENTS

ANTIPSYCHOTICS (NEUROLEPTICS)

Indications: Schizophrenia, schizophreniform disorder, schizoaffective disorder, mood disorders with psychotic features, bipolar disorder with psychotic features, major depression with psychotic features. Drug induced psychoses, organic psychoses, acute mania.

SIDE EFFECTS:

Akathesia: Restlessness, fidgeting, feeling a constant need to move about.

Dystonia: Involuntary muscular contractions, rigidity and cramping; frequently involves the jaw muscles as well as muscles in the neck, tongue, face and back, usually occurs in first weeks of therapy.

Neuroleptic Malignant Syndrome (NMS): Rigidity, delirium, fever, hyperthermia, sweating, hypotension, tachycardia and arrhythmias. Medication should be discontinued immediately. The fatality rate of neuromuscular syndrome is 20-30%. Treatment is dantrolene or bromocriptine.

Drug-Induced Parkinsonism: Rigidity beginning in shoulders and then spreading to the rest of the body; stooped posture, drooling, masked face, tremor of the jaw, tongue and upper extremities, akinesia.

Anti-Parkinsonism drugs used to treat extrapyramidal effects of neuroleptics:

Amantadine (Symmetrel) 100 mg, PO bid or tid
Benztropine (Cogentin) 1-2 mg, PO bid
Biperiden (Akineton) 1-3 mg, PO tid/qid
Diphenhydramine (Benadryl) 25 mg, PO bid/qid
Trihexyphenidyl (Artane, Tremin) 1-3 mg, PO bid/tid

Tardive Dyskinesia: Occurs with long-term use. Symptoms include tic-like movements of tongue, face and neck muscles, chewing movements, protrusion of tongue, excessive blinking and grimacing. Medication should be stopped if possible. No effective treatment exists.

Other Side Effects: Increased appetite, weight gain, photosensitivity, sedation, dry mouth, constipation, lowered seizure threshold, blurred vision, inhibition of ejaculation, skin rashes, EKG changes, reduced libido, cholestatic jaundice, agranulocytosis, hyperthermia, hypotension.

Drug Interactions: CNS depression with all CNS depressants. Absorption of Antipsychotics may be reduced by antacids.

ANTIPSYCHOTICS

BUTYROPHENONES

Haloperidol (Haldol)

Indications: Psychotic disorders, Tourette's syndrome.
Dosage Forms: 0,.5, 1, 2, 5, 10, 20 mg tabs, 2 mg/ml concentrate, 1 ml amp, 10 ml vial, 1 ml syringe, 5 mg/ml parenteral.
Dosage: 0.5-5 mg IM q4-8h prn or 0.5-5 mg PO bid/tid max 100 mg/day.
Sedation: Mild to moderate
Anticholinergic Effects: Less common
Hypotension: Less common
Extrapyramidal Effects: Very common

Droperidol (Inapsine)

Indications: Sedation, psychosis
Dosage Forms: 2.5 mg/ml amps; 2.5 mg/ml vial.
Dosage: 2.5-10 mg IV/IM.
Sedation: Moderate
Anticholinergic Effects: Less common

Dibenzazepine

Loxapine (Loxitane, Daxolin)

Indications: Psychosis
Dosage Forms: 5,10,25,50 mg tabs, 25 mg/ml concentrate, 1 ml/10 ml vial, 50 mg/ml parenteral.
Dosage: Adults: 12.5-50 mg IM q4-6h or 10-50 mg PO bid/tid max 250mg/day.
Sedation: Moderate
Anticholinergic Effects: Less common
Hypotension: Less common
Extrapyramidal Effects More common

Dihydroindolone

Molindone hydrochloride, (Molindone, Moban)

Indications: Psychotic disorders

Dosage Forms: 5, 10, 25, 50, 100 mg tabs; 20 mg/ml concentrate.

Dosage: Adults: 5-25 mg PO tid-qid max 225 mg/day.

Side Effects: Molindone is less likely to precipitate weight gain and should be considered in non-compliant patients who are concerned with weight.

Sedation: Moderate to high

Anticholinergic Effects: Less common

Hypotension: Less common

Extrapyramidal Effects: More common

Diphenylbutylpiperidine

Pimozide (Orap)

Indications: Tourette's syndrome

Dosage Forms: 2 mg tab.

Dosage: 1-2 mg PO qd; max 10 mg/day.

Side Effects: Increased occurrence of cardiac affects, galactorrhea, amenorrhea, dysmenorrhea.

Sedation: Moderate

Anticholinergic Effects: Less common

Hypotension: More common

Extrapyramidal Effects: More common

PHENOTHIAZINES:

Aliphatics

Chlorpromazine (Thorazine)

Indications: Psychotic disorders

Available in: 10, 25, 50, 100, 200 mg caps; 30, 100 mg/ml concentrate; 10 mg/5 ml syrup; 25, 100 mg Supp; 25 mg/ml amp.

Dosage: Adults: 10-50 mg PO/IM bid/tid/qid.

Side Effects: More likely to cause hypotension, agranulocytosis, allergic reactions.

Sedation: High

Anticholinergic Effects: More common

Hypotension: More common

Extrapyramidal Effects More common

Promazine (Sparine)

Used to Treat: Psychotic disorders, however, sparine has weak antipsychotic effects and is not a first line treatment.

Dosage Forms: 20 mg tabs.

Dosage: 10-200 mg PO/IM q4-6h max 1 g/day.

Side Effects: Allergic reactions; most common in persons with asthma.

Sedation: Moderate

Anticholinergic Effects: Less common

Hypotension: More common

Extrapyramidal Effects: Moderate

PIPERADINES:

Thioridazine (Mellaril)

Indications: Psychotic disorders, anxiety.

Dosage Forms: 10, 15, 25, 50, 100, 150, 200 mg tabs, 25 and 100 mg/ml sus; 30 mg/ml, 100 mg/ml concentrate.

Dosage: Adults: 25-100 mg PO tid; max 800 mg/day.

Side Effects: Retrograde ejaculation, more likely to cause hypotension, agranulocytosis, retinal injury.

Sedation: High

Hypotension: More common

Extrapyramidal Effects: Less common

Mesoridazine (Serentil)

Indications: Psychosis, organic brain syndrome.

Dosage Forms: 10, 25, 50, 100 mg tabs; 25 mg/ml concentrate; 25 mg/ml amp.

Dosage: 25-100 mg IM, 25-100 mg PO tid; max 400 mg/day .

Sedation: Moderate
Anticholinergic Effects: More common
Hypotension: More common
Extrapyramidal Effects: More common

PIPERAZINES:

Fluphenazine HCL (Prolixin) and Fluphenazine Decanote

Indications: Psychotic disorders.
Dosage Forms: 1, 2.5, 5, 10 mg tabs, 5 mg/ml concentrate; 2.5 mg/ml parenteral; 2.5 mg/5ml elixir.
Dosage: Fluphenazine HCL, 1.25 mg IM q6-8h; max 10 mg/day **OR** 2.5-10 mg PO day (divided doses), max 40 mg/day; elderly/adolescents: 1-2.5 mg daily. Fluphenazine decanote, 12.5 - 25 mg IM q 2-4 weeks max 100 mg/day.
Sedation: Moderate
Anticholinergic Effects: Less common
Hypotension: Less common
Extrapyramidal Effects: More common

Perphenazine (Trilafon)

Indications: Psychosis
Dosage Forms: 2,4,8,16 mg tabs; 16 mg/5 ml concentrate; 5 mg/ml amps.
Dosage: 8-16 mg PO bid-qid max 64 mg/day or 5 mg IM q6h max 30 mg/day.
Side Effects: Perphenazine contains sodium bisulfite which may precipitate asthma attacks and allergic reactions.
Sedation: Moderate
Anticholinergic Effects: Less common
Hypotension: More common
Extrapyramidal Effects: More common

Trifluoperazine (Stelazine)

Indications: Psychotic disorders.
Available in 1, 2, 5, 10 mg tabs; 10 mg/ml concentrate; 10 ml vial; 2 mg/ml parenteral.
Dosage: 1-2 mg IM q4-6h max 10 mg/day, 2-5 mg PO bid; max 40 mg/day.
Sedation: Moderate

Anticholinergic Effects: More common
Hypotension: Less common
Extrapyramidal Effects: More common

Prochlorperazine (Compazine)

Indications: Antiemetic
Dosage Forms: 5,10,25 mg tabs; 5 mg/ml syrup; 10 ml vial; 1,2 ml syringe; 2.5, 5, 25 mg supp; 2 ml amp; 5 mg/ml Paternal.
Dosage: 5-10 mg PO tid/qid; 100 mg/day max, 10-20 mg IM q4-6h.
Side Effects: Precipitation of asthma attacks.
Sedation: Moderate
Anticholinergic Effects: Less common
Extrapyramidal Effects: High

THIOXANTHENES

Chlorprothixene (Taractan)

Indications: Psychotic disorders, behavioral disorders in mentally retarded.
Dosage Forms: 10, 25, 50, 100 mg tabs; 100 mg / 5 mg concentrate; 25 mg/2ml amp.
Dosage: 25-50 mg PO/IM tid/qid.
Side Effects: Inhibits motor coordination, may cause allergic reactions (most common in patients with a history of allergic reactions to aspirin).
Sedation: High
Anticholinergic Effects Less common
Hypotension: More common
Extrapyramidal Effects: Moderate

Thiothixene (Navane)

Indications: Psychotic disorders
Dosage Forms: 1, 2, 5, 10, 20 mg caps; 5 mg/ml concentrate; 2 mg vial; 2, 5 mg/ml parenteral.
Dosage: 2-5 mg PO tid, 2-5 mg q6-12h IM; max 30 mg/day.
Sedation: High

Anticholinergic Effects Less common

Hypotension: Less common

Extrapyramidal Effects: More common

OTHER ANTIPSYCHOTICS:

Clozapine (Clozaril)

Indications: Refractory schizophrenia

Dosage Forms: 25,100 mg tabs.

Dosage: 25 mg qd/bid increase by 25-50 mg/day to 300-600 mg day; max 900 mg/day.

Side effects: Clozapine does not cause extrapyramidal side effects. Agranulocytosis, seizures, orthostatic hypertension, sedation, GI distress, tachycardia, fever, anticholinergic effects, cognitive impairment.

Contraindications: Granulocytopenia, myeloproliferative disorders.

Interactions: Potentiation of antihypertensive medications.

TRICYCLIC ANTIDEPRESSANTS

Indications for use: Major depression, bipolar disorder, psychotic depression with antipsychotic, panic disorder, agoraphobia with panic attacks, bulimia, organic mood syndrome, enuresis, dysthymia, schizoaffective disorder.

SIDE EFFECTS:

Anticholinergic Effects: Constipation, dry mouth, blurred vision, urinary hesitancy, heat intolerance.

Cardiac Effects: EKG changes, T-wave flattening, prolonged PR and QT interval, tachycardia; contraindicated in patients with bi-fascicular block, prolonged QT interval and left bundle branch block.

Autonomic Effects:

Ejaculatory dysfunction, impotence, sweating, blurred vision, dysuria.

Other Side Effects Lowering of seizure threshold; anorexia, nausea, vomiting, weight gain; insomnia, constipation; orthostatic hypotension, restlessness, sedation. Bipolar patients treated with TCA's may become manic. Elderly patients require lower doses.

Drug Interactions: CNS depression with other CNS depressants, sedatives, antihistamines or antipsychotics, alcohol, and antipsychotics. Hypertensive crisis with MAO inhibitors. TCA plasma levels are increased by amphetamines, acetazolamide, antipsychotics, disulfiram, exogenous thyroid hormone, glucocorticoids, oral contraceptives, salicylates or thiazides.

TCA plasma levels are decreased by alcohol, barbiturates, carbamazepine, cigarette smoking, phenobarbital, phenytoin, primadone and rifampin. Hypotension is worsened by beta-blockers, clonidine and diuretics. Effects of warfarin increased. Levodopa absorption may be depressed.

CYCLIC COMPOUNDS

Amitriptyline (Elavil)

Indications: Depression (especially endogenous).
Dosage Forms: 10, 25, 50, 75, 100, 150 mg tabs; 10 mg/ml inj.
Dosage: 25-200 mg PO qd, max 300 mg/day.

Amoxapine (Asendin)

Indications: Psychotic, endogenous depressions, anxiety and agitation with accompanying depression.
Dosage Forms: 25, 50, 75 mg tabs.
Dosage: 150 mg PO qd OR 50 mg bid/tid, Elderly/Adolescents: 25-100 mg PO qd, max 225 mg/day.
Time delay for therapeutic effect: Two to six weeks.

Desipramine (Norpramin)

Indications: Depression (especially endogenous).
Dosage Forms: 10, 25, 50, 75, 100, 150 mg tablets; 25, 50 mg capsules.
Dosage: 25-75 mg PO qhs, increase to a max of 300 mg/day.
Elderly: 25-100 mg; max 150 mg/day.
Time delay for therapeutic effect: 2 to 6 weeks

Doxepin (Adapin, Sinequan)

Indications: Depression.
Dosage Forms: 15, 25, 50, 75, 100, 150 mg caps; 10 mg ml liq.
Dosage: 25-75 mg PO qd, increase gradually to a max of 300 mg/day.

Imipramine (Tofranil)

Indications: Depression (especially endogenous), enuresis.
Dosage Forms: 10, 25, 50, 75, 100, 125, 150 mg tabs; 25/2 ml inj.
Time delay for therapeutic affect: One to six weeks.
Dosage: 25-75 mg PO qhs increase to a max of 300 mg/day. Elderly: 30-40 mg PO qhs, max 100 mg.

Maprotiline (Ludiomil)

Indications: Dysthymic disorder, bipolar disorder, depression.
Dosage Forms: 25, 50, 75 mg tabs.
Dosage: 25-75 mg PO qd increase to a max of 225 mg, Elderly: 25-75 mg PO qd.
Contraindications: Patients with liver disease or epilepsy.

Nortriptyline (Pamelor)

Indications: Depression (especially endogenous).
Dosage Forms: 10, 25, 50, 75 mg; 10 mg/5 mg liq.
Dosage: 25-100 mg PO qd, max 150 mg, Elderly: 30-50 mg daily in divided doses.

Protriptyline (Vivactil)

Indications: Depression
Dosage Forms: 5, 10 mg tabs
Dosage: 5-10 mg PO tid max 60 mg/day.

Trimipramine (Surmontil)

Indications: Depression (Endogenous).
Dosage Forms: 25, 50, 100 mg caps.
Delay for therapeutic affect: One to four weeks
Dosage: 25 mg PO tid max 300 mg/day.

NEWER ANTIDEPRESSANTS

Prozac (Fluoxetine hydrochloride)

Indications: Depression

Time delay for therapeutic effect: Four to five weeks.

Dosage Forms: 20 mg tabs.

Dosage: 20 mg PO qd, max 80 mg.

Side effects: Restlessness, insomnia, rash, CNS stimulation, headache, anorexia and weight loss, impaired motor performance, anxiety, seizures, nausea, diarrhea. If restlessness is a problem combine with .25-0.5 mg clonazepam bid. Insomnia: reduce dose or add 25-50 mg trazodone PO qhs.

Contraindications : Discontinue if rash develops; pregnancy or lactation.

Interactions: Hypertensive crises with MAO inhibitors, CNS stimulation with tryptophan; seizures with diazepam.

Trazodone (Desyrel)

Indications: Major depression

Dosage Forms: 50, 100, 150, 300 mg tabs.

Dosage: 50 mg PO bid/tid; increase by 50 mg every 3-4 days, max 400 mg/day.

Side Effects: fatigue, lightheadedness, headache, insomnia, GI upset, orthostatic hypotension.

Bupropion (Wellbutrin)

Indications Depression.

Dosage Forms: 75, 100 mg tabs.

Dosage: 100 mg PO tid, max 150 mg per dose with at least 4 hrs between doses to prevent seizures.

Side Effects Anxiety, agitation, restlessness, insomnia, headache diarrhea, nausea.

MONAMINE OXIDASE INHIBITORS

Indications: Atypical depression, major depression, dysthymic disorder, panic attacks, agoraphobia with panic attacks.

Side Effects: Orthostatic hypotension, anxiety, headache, Insomnia, impotence, dry mouth, agitation, edema, dizziness, constipation, weight gain, seizures, GI upset. Manic episodes may occur in patients with bipolar disorder; psychosis may occur in patients with schizophrenia.

Hypertensive Crises: Occurs with other antidepressants, tyramine containing foods, adrenergic medications. Patients should be instructed to avoid substances that precipitate a crises. Symptoms of hypertensive crises: Headache, diaphoresis, mydriasis, hypertension, neck stiffness, photophobia, tachycardia.

Contraindications: Cardiovascular, renal or liver disease, pheochromocytoma, severe hypertension.

Foods Which Precipitate Hypertensive Crises:

Fruits: Canned figs, any over ripe fruit.

Vegetables: Fava beans (Italian green beans), sauerkraut, avocados.

Dairy: Aged yogurt, strong cheeses.

Meat: Liver, spoiled meat, fermented sausages (bologna, salami, pepperoni).

Fish: Dried, salted fish; pickled or dried herring, caviar.

Beverages: Beer, chianti wine, red wine, any non-distilled alcohol.

Drug Interactions

Drugs Which Precipitate Hypertensive Crises: Amphetamines, cocaine, dopamine, L-dopa, methyldopa, phenylephrine, pseudoephedrine (Sudafed), metaraminol, ephedrine, epinephrine, phenylpropanolamine, norepinephrine.

Isocarboxazid (Marplan)

Indications: Depressed patients who are refractory to tricyclic antidepressants or ECT, or when tricyclic antidepressants are contraindicated.

Dosage Forms: 10 mg tabs.

Dosage: 15 mg PO qd/bid increase to 60 mg/day; max 90 mg/day.

Phenelzine (Nardil)

Indications: Atypical, non-endogenous or neurotic depression; depressions with phobic, anxiety features.

Dosage Forms: 15 mg tabs

Dosage: 15 mg PO tid, increase as needed to 30 mg PO tid; max, 60 mg/day.

Tranylcypromine (Pamate)

Indications: Major depression.

Dosage Forms: 10 mg tabs.

Dosage: 10 mg PO tid, increase as needed by 10 mg every other week; max 60 mg.

BENZODIAZEPINES

Indications: Insomnia, alcohol withdrawal, panic attacks, generalized anxiety disorder, seizure disorders.

Side Effects: Sedation, impaired concentration, drowsiness; tolerance, dependence, rash, hypotension, agitation.

Symptoms of Withdrawal: Insomnia, tremor, agitation, abdominal discomfort, photosensitivity, seizures and psychosis.

Drug Interactions: Alcohol, disulfiram, valproic acid and Isoniazid all reduce the metabolism of benzodiazepines. Estrogens and rifampin increase the metabolism of benzodiazepines. Antacids lower absorption, and alcohol increases absorption.

Overdose Symptoms: Ataxia, hypotonia, nystagmus, excessive sedation and coma.

Treatment: Supportive care

Note: Elderly patients may require lower doses: Diazepam, prazepam, chlorazepate, chlordiazepoxide are long acting agents and may be given less frequently than short acting agents (alprazolam, halazepam, oxazepam, and lorazepam).

Alprazolam (Xanax)

Indications: Anxiety disorders.

Dosage Forms: 0.25, 0.5, 1, 2 mg tabs.

Dosage: 0.25-0.5 mg PO tid; elderly 0.25 bid/tid; max 4mg/day.

Chlordiazepoxide (Librium)

Indications: Anxiety disorders, acute alcohol withdrawal.
Dosage Forms: 5, 10, 25 mg tabs; 100 mg/2 ml (Amp).
Dosage: 5-25 mg PO tid; alcohol withdrawal 25-100 mg PO q2-4h; elderly 5 mg bid/tid/qid; max 300 mg/day.

Clorazepate (Tranxene)

Indications: Anxiety, alcohol withdrawal
Dosage Forms: 3.75 mg, 7.5 mg, 15 mg, scored tabs.
Dosage: 10 mg PO tid, increase as needed to a max of 90 mg/day; elderly: 7.5-15 mg daily in divided doses.

Diazepam (Valium)

Indications: Anxiety, acute alcohol withdrawal.
Dosage Forms: 2.5, 10 mg, scored tabs; 5 mg/ml inj.
Dosage: 2-10 mg PO bid/qid; elderly 2-2.5 mg qd/bid.

Flurazepam (Dalmane)

Indications: Insomnia
Dosage Forms: 15, 30 mg tabs
Dosage: 15-30 mg PO qhs.

Lorazepam (Ativan)

Indications: Anxiety
Dosage Forms: 0.5, 1, 2 mg tabs
Dosage: 0.5-1.0 mg bid/tid; elderly: 1-2 mg/day in divided doses; max 10 mg/day.

Oxazepam (Serax)

Indications: Anxiety disorders, depressive disorders with anxiety, alcohol withdrawal.
Dosage Forms: 10, 15, 30 mg caps; 15 mg tabs.

Dosage: 10-15 mg PO tid/qid; elderly: 10 mg PO tid/qid.
Alcohol withdrawal: 15-30 mg PO tid/qid.

Prazepam (Centrax)

Indications: Anxiety disorders.
Dosage Forms: 5, 10, 20 mg cap; 15 mg tabs.
Dosage: 10 mg PO tid; elderly: 10-15 mg daily in divided doses; max 60 mg/day.

Quazepam (Doral)

Indications: Insomnia
Dosage Forms 7.5, 15 mg tabs.
Dosage: 15 mg PO qhs; elderly: 7.5 mg PO qhs.

Temazepam (Restoril)

Indications: Insomnia
Dosage Forms: 15, 30 mg caps
Dosage: 15-30 mg PO qhs; elderly: 15 mg PO qhs.

Triazolam (Halcion)

Indications: Insomnia
Dosage Forms: 0.125, 0.25 mg tabs
Dosage: 0.125-0.25 mg PO qhs, max 0.25 mg; elderly or debilitated .125 mg.

OTHER ANTIANXIETY AGENTS

Buspirone (Buspar)

Indications: Anxiety, generalized anxiety disorder.
Dosage Forms: 5, 10 mg tabs.
Usual daily dose: Adults 5-10 mg PO tid/qid; max 60 mg/day.
Side Effects: Less sedating than other antianxiety agents, drowsiness, headache, dizziness, insomnia, fatigue, GI upset, tachycardia, angina,

palpitations, hair loss, rash, nausea, pruritus, dry skin, amenorrhea, thyroid abnormalities.

Interactions: Hypertensive crises with MAOI's; fluoxetine decreases effects of buspirone, potentiation of haloperidol, elevation of serum ALT when taken in conjunction with trazodone.

PSYCHOSTIMULANTS

Dextroamphetamine (Dexedrine)

Indications: Narcolepsy, attention deficit hyperactivity disorder, depression.

Dosage Forms: 5 mg tabs; 5 mg/ml elixir, 10 mg caps.

Dosage: 5 mg PO qd/bid; children with attention deficit hyperactivity disorder: 3-5 years: 2.5 mg daily; over 6 years: 5 mg PO qd/bid; over 12 years: 10 mg PO qd.

Side effects: CNS stimulation, hypertension, tachycardia, dry mouth, GI upset, urticaria, anorexia.

Contraindications: Cardiovascular disease, glaucoma, hyperthyroidism, hypertension; history of drug or alcohol abuse.

Interactions: Hypertensive crises with MAO inhibitors; tricyclic antidepressants increase potency of dextroamphetamine; potentiation of phenobarbital, norepinephrine, meperidine, and phenytoin. Inhibits effects of ethosuximide, adrenergic blockers.

Methamphetamine (Desoxyn)

Indications: Attention deficit disorder.

Dosage Forms: 5 mg tabs; 5, 10, 15 mg sustained release tabs.

Dosage: Over 6 years: 5 mg qd/bid, increase weekly by 5 mg daily to 20-25 mg, max.

Side effects: CNS stimulation, palpitations, hypertension, dry mouth, urticaria, anorexia, insomnia, GI disturbances, psychosis.

Contraindications: Cardiovascular disease, hypertension, hyperthyroidism, glaucoma, Tourette's Syndrome.

Interactions: Hypertensive crisis with MAO inhibitors, increased effect with tricyclic antidepressants.

Methylphenidate (Ritalin)

Indications: Narcolepsy, attention deficit disorder.
Dosage Forms: 5, 10, 20 mg tabs; 5 mg/ml elixir.
Dosage: 5 mg PO bid increase up to 60 mg day divided doses; children: over 6 years: 5 mg PO bid increase weekly, max 60 mg/day.
Side effects: Insomnia, CNS stimulation, anorexia, hypertension, cardiac arrhythmias, psychosis, seizures, rash, blood dyscrasias, alopecia.
Contraindications: Glaucoma, family history of Tourette's syndrome.
Interactions: Increased effects with MAO inhibitors, pressor agents; increases effect of anticonvulsants, anticoagulants, tricyclic antidepressants.

Pemoline (Cylert)

Indications: Attention deficit disorder.
Dosage Forms: 18.75, 37.5, 75 mg tabs; 37.5 mg chewable tabs.
Dosage: Children: over 6 years: 37.5 mg increased weekly by 18.75 mg, max 112.5 mg daily.
Side effects: CNS stimulation, anorexia, insomnia, hepatic dysfunction, abdominal pain, nausea, depression, headache, dizziness, lowered seizure threshold.
Contraindications: Psychosis, anxiety, impaired hepatic function, Tourette's Syndrome.
Interactions: Increased affect with CNS stimulants.

LITHIUM CARBONATE

Indications: Bipolar disorder, mania, cyclothymia; possibly effective in schizoaffect ive disorder.
Dosage: Starting dose 300 mg PO tid, increase dose based on blood level (usual range is 1.2-1.4 meq/L).
Side Effects:
Central Nervous System: Headache, transient weakness, lethargy, mental dullness, slurred speech.
Tremor: Treat by decreasing dose and if necessary, add propranolol 20-60 mg

per day starting at 10-20 mg bid and increasing prn, or use atenolol 50 mg per day.

Gastrointestinal Side Effects: Diarrhea, nausea, anorexia, bloating, cramps, abdominal pain.

Endocrine Side Effects: Hypothyroidism, hyperparathyroidism, goiter; hyperglycemia. Check thyroid function tests at least once every six months.

Renal Side Effects: Thirst, polyuria, polydipsia; diabetes insipidus which can be treated with hydrochlorothiazide 50 mg daily. Rare side effects include nephrotic syndrome and an acute rise in serum creatinine.

Cardiac Side Effects: Myocarditis, heart block, T wave flattening, arrhythmias, edema.

Dermatologic Side Effects: Folliculitis, acne, psoriasis; rarely alopecia and exfoliative dermatitis.

Other Side Effects: Leukocytosis, weakness, rash, weight gain.

Contraindications: Pregnancy and lactation, history of myocardial infarction.

Drug Interactions: Lithium levels may increase with thiazides, acetazolamide, furosemide, erythromycin and methyldopa. Lithium levels may be lowered by calcium channel, blockers, valproic acid. Confusional states and sedation may be produced by antipsychotics. Renal toxicity has been reported with the combination of metronidazole and lithium.

Lab & Blood Levels: Draw blood twelve hours after last oral dose, therapeutic range is 0.6-1.5 mEq/l . Monitor blood count, BUN, creatinine, urinalysis, thyroid function tests; ECG for patients over 40.

ANTICONVULSANTS IN PSYCHIATRY

Carbamazepine (Tegretol)

Indications: Bipolar disorder, atypical depression.

Dosage Forms 100, 200 mg tabs

Dosage 200 mg bid increased weekly to 800-1200 mg/day.

Side Effects Nausea, vomiting, blurred vision, drowsiness, dizziness, ataxia. Leukopenia, aplastic anemia, thrombocytopenia and hepatic hypersensitivity.

Contraindications Pregnancy

Interactions Decrease in serum levels of clonazepam, valproic acid, haloperidol, phenytoin. Phenobarbital, primidone and phenytoin decrease carbamazepine levels. Erythromycin, isoniazid, and propoxyphene increase carbamazepine levels.

Clonazepam (Klonopin)

Indications Panic disorder, generalized anxiety disorder.
Dosage Forms 0.5, 1, 2 mg tabs.
Dosage 0.5 mg PO tid increased by 0.5 mg to 1-2 mg qd/tid.
Side effects Sedation
Contraindications: Narrow angle glaucoma, liver disease.

Valproic Acid (Depakene) and Divalproex (Depakote)

Indications: Acute mania, prevention of mania.
Dosage Forms: Depakene: 250 mg caps. Depakote: 125,250,500 mg tabs.
Dosage: 250 mg PO bid/tid, increase as tolerated to blood level of 40-100 mcg/ml.
Side Effects: Elevations in aminotransferase, hepatitis, GI upset, weight gain, drowsiness, sedation, dizziness, dysarthria, ataxia, tremor, bone marrow depression, thrombocytopenia, pancreatitis, alopecia.
Contraindications: Liver disease.
Interactions: Increase in effects of MAOI's, decrease in effects of carbamazepine.

OTHER AGENTS

Amobarbital (Amytal)

Indications: Hypnosis, insomnia, sedation
Dosage Forms: 15, 30, 50, 100 mg tabs; 65, 200 mg caps; 44 mg/5 ml conc.
Dosage: 15-50 mg PO bid/tid OR 50-200 mg PO qhs.
Side Effects: CNS depression, drowsiness, nausea, vomiting, cramping, diarrhea, dependence, withdrawal (titrate gradually), nightmares.
Contraindications: Acute intermittent porphyria, respiratory impairment.
Interactions: CNS depression with CNS depressants.

Meprobamate (Equanil, Miltown)

Indication: Sedation
Dosage Forms: 200, 400, 600 mg tabs.
Dosage: 1.2-1.6 g/day in four divided doses.
Side Effects: Drowsiness, CNS depression, nausea, vomiting, cramping, diarrhea, dependence, withdrawal (titrate gradually), nightmares.

Contraindications: Acute intermittent porphyria, respiratory impairment.
Interactions: CNS depression with CNS depressants.

Benztropine (Cogentin)

Indications Neuroleptic induced parkinsonism, dystonic reactions.
Dosage Forms: 1, 2 mg tabs; 1 mg/ml ampules.
Dosage: 1-2 mg PO bid/tid OR 1-2 mg IM; max 8 mg/day.
Side effects: Dry mouth, blurred vision, nausea, weakness, confusion, constipation, rapid pulse.
Interactions Increase anticholinergic effects with other anticholinergics.

Biperiden (Akineton)

Indications Neuroleptic induced parkinsonism, dystonic reactions.
Dosage Forms: 2 mg tabs, 1 mg/ml parenteral.
Dosage: 2 mg PO qd-tid OR 2 mg IM/IV; max 6 mg/day.
Side Effects: Constipation, impaired memory and concentration.
Interactions Increase anticholinergic effects with other anticholinergics.

Trihexyphenidyl (Artane)

Indications Neuroleptic induced parkinsonism, dystonic reactions.
Dosage Forms: 2, 5 mg tabs; 5 mg caps.
Dosage: 5 mg qd-tid.
Side Effects: Blurred vision, dry mouth, constipation, nausea, vomiting, tachycardia, weakness, urinary retention, restlessness, agitation.
Interactions: Increased anticholinergic effects with other anticholinergics.

BETA-BLOCKERS AND OTHER AGENTS

Atenolol (Tenormin)

Indications: Akathisia, lithium induced tremor.
Dosage Forms 50, 100 mg tabs.
Dosage: 50 mg PO qd, max 200 mg.
Side Effects: Depression, fatigue, dizziness, GI upset, hypertension, bradycardia, rashes, dyspnea, impotence, insomnia, nightmares.

Contraindications: Cardiac dysfunction (arrhythmias, AV block, sinus bradycardia) hyperthyroidism, asthma.
Interactions: Ampicillin, aluminum salts, NSAIDs decrease therapeutic effects of atenolol; Effects if warfarin may be increased, increase in half life of antipyrine, when nifedipine is taken in conjunction with atenolol both are potentiated; increased effects of lidocaine and insulin; hydralazine and cimetidine increase effects, increased hypotension with antipsychotics and other hypotensives.

Propanolol (Inderal)

Indications: Anxiety, akathisia, lithium induced tremor.
Dosage Forms: 10, 20, 40, 60, 80, 90 mg tabs; 60, 80, 120, 160 mg caps; 20 mg/5ml, 40 mg/5ml oral liq.
Dosage: 20-40 mg qd-tid.
Side Effects: Diarrhea, nausea, vomiting, dizziness, irritability, insomnia, nightmares, depression, weakness, GI upset, fatigue,hypotension, eosinophilia, elevations of serum aminotransferase and serum creatinine, hypotension, bradycardia, impotence,
Contraindications: Impaired cardiac function, diabetes, asthma, Reynaud's disease.
Interactions: Increased effects of lidocaine and insulin; hydralazine and cimetidine increase effects of propranolol, increased hypotension with antipsychotics.
Carbamazepine, barbiturates, cholestyramine, NSAID's, rifampin and salicylates may decrease effectiveness of propranolol; hypertensive crises with MAOI's.

Disulfiram (Antabuse)

Indications: Alcoholism
Dosage Forms: 250, 500 mg tabs.
Dosage: 250-500 mg PO qd.
Side Effects: Fatigue, headache, impotence, acne, rash, irritability, insomnia, confusion, hepatitis, and less commonly: Peripheral neuropathy, delirium and psychosis. If alcohol is consumed, headache, nausea, vomiting, pallor, thirst, diaphoresis, chest pain, anxiety, blurred vision, respiratory depression, arrhythmias, heart failure, seizures and death may occur. The more serious

side effects are in patient taking over 500 mg daily.

Contraindication: Cardiovascular disease, psychosis, alcohol intoxication.

Interactions:

-Severe adverse reaction with alcohol consumption.

-Anticoagulant effects are increased when they are administered in conjunction with disulfiram.

-Theophylline is potentiated.

-Metronidazole may precipitate a psychotic episode when it is administered in conjunction with disulfiram.

-Perphenazine effects and levels are decreased.

-Phenytoin levels are increase significantly.

-CNS depression may occur when disulfiram is taken in conjunction with benzodiazepines.

-Isoniazid may cause behavioral changes.

-Tricyclics may cause organic brain syndrome when they are taken in conjunction with disulfiram.

ELECTROCONVULSIVE THERAPY

Indications: Major depression, bipolar disorder, schizoaffective disorder, catatonic schizophrenia, catatonia.

Side Effects: Mild amnesia, EEG changes, transient cardiac arrhythmias,dizziness, confusion, myalgias, nausea, headaches, transient hypertension or hypotension.

Contraindications: Myocardial infarction, increased intracranial pressure.

Relative Contraindications: Severe cardiovascular, liver or pulmonary disease, recent cerebrovascular accident, intracranial mass, severe hypertension.

Pre-ECT Evaluation: Complete medical workup and history including cardiac and neurologic status; chest and spine x-rays, ECG.

Administration of ECT: Remove dentures. Administer glycopyrolate or atropine to reduce secretions, then a short acting barbiturate, methohexital (40-80 mg) is given. Oxygen is administered via endotracheal tube by bag & mask, and a muscle relaxants (succinylcholine 40-80 mg) is given. Electrodes are placed unilaterally or bilaterally, 12 or more centimeters apart. Current is administered at a for a duration of 0.5 seconds and 140-150 volts.

To Order Additional Copies

Current Clinical Strategies, Manual of HIV/AIDS Therapy By Laurance Pieperl, MD., University of California, San Francisco	#___ x $8.75
Current Clinical Strategies, MEDICINE, Paul D. Chan, NEW 1992 edition	#___ x $8.75
Current Clinical Strategies, GYNECOLOGY & OBSTETRICS	#___ x $8.75
Current Clinical Strategies, PEDIATRICS	#___ x $8.75
FAMILY MEDICINE Pediatrics, Medicine, Gynecology, Obstetrics	#___ x $26.25
DIAGNOSTIC HISTORY & PHYSICAL EXAMINATION in MEDICINE	#___ x $8.75
Current Clinical Strategies, PSYCHIATRY* Lisa Burwell-Sipes	#___ x $8.75
Handbook of Psychiatric Drug Therapy Lisa Burwell-Sipes	#___ x $8.75
OUTPATIENT MEDICINE	#___ x $8.75
CRITICAL CARE MEDICINE (available October 1992)	#___ x $8.75
Current Clinical Strategies, SURGERY (available February 1993)	#___ x $8.75
	Total ______

Prices are in US dollars & include shipping; Canada, $10.75; UK, £4.00; Australia, $9.75. Other countries, send check in US dollars. Prices and availability subject to change without notice.
Phone: 714-721-0710.

Send order & check payable to:

Current Clinical Strategies Publishing
4200 Park Newport Avenue, Suite 214;
Newport Beach, California, USA 92660-6025

Return Address: ________________________________

Check if Resident or Student _____

Is this book sold at your local medical book store? ___ yes ___ no

Have you contacted this store and suggested that they begin to carry this book? ___ yes ___ no

Name of bookstore: ________________________________

Please complete reverse side.

Dear Reader,

Thank you for purchasing this copy of Current Clinical Strategies. If you have suggestions or comments, please contact the publisher at the address below. Readers are also encouraged to write additional sections or to submit their own manuscripts for publication. Acknowledgement and remuneration may be provided.

If this book is not available in your local bookstore, please contact them and suggest that they carry this line of books, and your next copy will be sent at half price.

Personalized and individually printed copies may be obtained free of charge. To receive a customized copy with individualized drug or treatment preferences, send modifications and recommendations to the address below.

Current Clinical Strategies Publishing International
4200 Park Newport, Suite 214; Newport Beach, California, 92660
FAX or Phone: 714-721-0710

Suggested additions, problems or criticisms: ______________________________

Dear Reader,

Thank you for purchasing this copy of Current Clinical Strategies. If you have suggestions or comments, please contact the publisher at the address below. Readers are also encouraged to write additional sections or to submit their own manuscripts for publication. Acknowledgement and remuneration may be provided.

If this book is not available in your local bookstore, please contact them and suggest that they carry this line of books, and your next copy will be sent at half price.

Personalized and individually printed copies may be obtained free of charge. To receive a customized copy with individualized drug or treatment preferences, send modifications and recommendations to the address below.

Current Clinical Strategies Publishing International
4200 Park Newport, Suite 214; Newport Beach, California, 92660
FAX or Phone: 714-721-0710

Suggested additions, problems or criticisms: ______________________